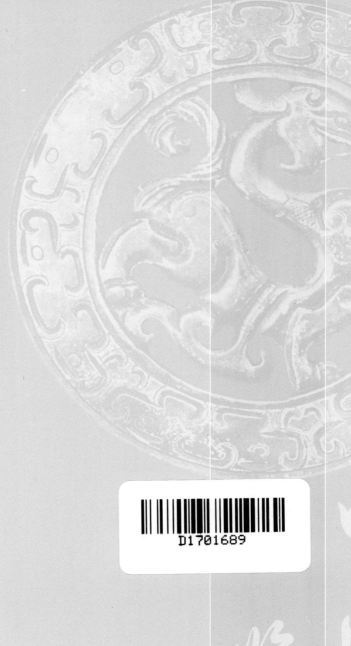
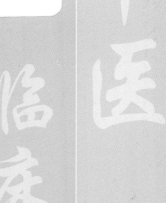

Sandra Collins
Heilpraktikerin
Sigmaringer Str. 1
D - 10713 Berlin

D1701689

The plant shown on the cover is Lycium chinese mill. In Chinese medicine, its dried ripe fruit is known as gŏu qī zĭ (Fructus Lycii), more commonly known as wolfberry fruit. Gŏu qī zĭ tonifies the liver and kidney, replenishes essence, and brightens the eyes. It is also commonly used in the treatment of alopecia due to patterns of kidney deficiency.

Project Editor: Liu Shui & Zeng Chun
Copy Editor: Cen Cong
Book Designer: Li Xi
Cover Designer: Li Xi
Typesetter: Wei Hong-bo

The Clinical Practice of Chinese Medicine

Acne & Alopecia

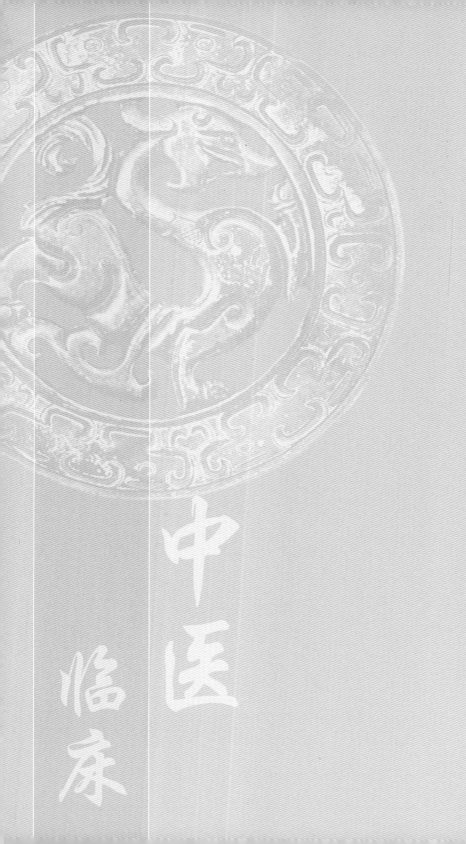

The Clinical Practice of Chinese Medicine
Acne & Alopecia

Fan Rui-qiang
Chief Physician & Professor of Chinese External Medicine, the Second Teaching Hospital of Guangzhou University of CM, Guangzhou, China

Xuan Guo-wei
Chief Physician & Professor of Chinese External Medicine, the Second Teaching Hospital of Guangzhou University of CM, Guangzhou, China

Contributors

Huang Yong-jing, M.S. TCM
Associate Chief Physician of Chinese External Medicine

Wu Wei, M.S. TCM
Attending Physician of Chinese External Medicine

Chen Da-can
Chief Physician & Professor of Chinese External Medicine

Hu Dong-liu, M.S. TCM
Associate Chief Physician of Chinese External Medicine

Chen Xiu-yang, M.S. TCM
Attending Physician of Chinese External Medicine

Translated by
Xu Zhen-zhen, M.S. TCM.
Wang Yan, M.S. TCM.
Wu Yuan-yuan, M.S. TCM.
Wang Dong, M.S. TCM.

Edited by **Therese Hui**, M.S. TCM, M.A., L.Ac.

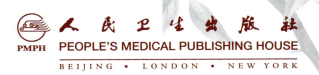

PEOPLE'S MEDICAL PUBLISHING HOUSE
BEIJING • LONDON • NEW YORK

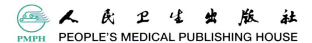

PEOPLE'S MEDICAL PUBLISHING HOUSE

Website: http://www.pmph.com

Book Title: The Clinical Practice of Chinese Medicine: **Acne & Alopecia**
中医临床实用系列：痤疮与脱发

Copyright © 2008 by People's Medical Publishing House. All rights reserved. No part of this publication may be reproduced, stored in a database or retrieval system, or transmitted in any form or by any electronic, mechanical, photocopy, or other recording means, without the prior written permission of the publisher.

Contact address: Bldg 3, 3 Qu, Fangqunyuan, Fangzhuang, Beijing 100078, P.R. China, phone/fax: 8610 6769 1034, E-mail: pmph@pmph.com

For text and trade sales, as well as review copy enquiries, please contact PMPH at pmphsales@gmail.com

---

Disclaimer

This book is for educational and reference purposes only. In view of the possibility of human error or changes in medical science, neither the author, editor, publisher, nor any other party who has been involved in the preparation or publication of this work guarantees that the information contained herein is in every respect accurate or complete. The medicinal therapy and treatment techniques presented in this book are provided for the purpose of reference only. If readers wish to attempt any of the techniques or utilize any of the medicinal therapies contained in this book, the publisher assumes no responsibility for any such actions.

It is the responsibility of the readers to understand and adhere to local laws and regulations concerning the practice of these techniques and methods. The authors, editors, and publishers disclaim all responsibility for any liability, loss, injury, or damage incurred as a consequence, directly or indirectly, of the use and application of any of the contents of this book.

First published: 2008
ISBN: 978-7-117-09888-5/R · 9889

Cataloguing in Publication Data:
A catalog record for this book is available from the CIP-Database China.

Printed in The People's Republic of China

About the Authors

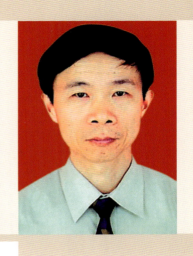

范瑞强　教授

Professor **Fan Rui-qiang** serves as a professor, chief physician, doctoral supervisor and academic disciplinary leader at the Second Teaching Hospital of Guangzhou University of Chinese Medicine.

A former director of the scientific research center and Chinese outpatient department at the Hongkong Yan Chai Hospital, Professor Fan now serves as the director of the dermatology department of Guangdong Provincial Hospital of TCM. He is an assistant director of the China Association for Traditional Chinese Medicine of Dermatology, assistant director of the STD Department of Dermatology and STD Board of China Association of Integrative Medicine. He is also a board member of the Specialty Committee of Chinese Medical Sexology of the China Sexology Association, member of the Specialty Committee of STD Prevention Board of China Sexology Association, and director of the Specialty Committee of Dermatology and STD of Guangdong Provincial Association of Integrative Medicine. He serves as the assistant director of the Specialty Committee of Dermatology of the Guangdong Provincial Chinese Medicine Association and assistant director of the Specialty Committee of Chinese Cosmetology of the Guangdong Provincial Chinese Medicine Association. In addition, he is also a member of the Guangdong Medical Association of Allergology. He has done thorough research on various skin diseases such as acne, dermatomycosis, STDs, lupus erythematosus and eczema.

Professor Fan was in charge of 23 national or ministry level projects and has won six scientific awards. He wrote *Selected Practical Empirical Formulae of Dermatology and STD* and was editor of several publications on dermatology. He has also written and edited nine other works and has published over 60 academic articles. He has been recognized as Guangdong Provincial Outstanding Youth Chinese Physician by the Ministry of Personnel of Guangdong, the Health Bureau of Guangdong Province and the State Administration of Traditional Chinese Medicine of the People's Republic of China.

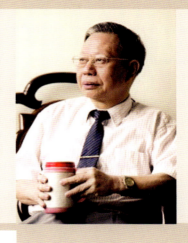

禤 国 维 教授

Professor **Xuan Guo-wei** serves as a professor, chief physician, and doctoral supervisor of the Guangzhou University of Chinese Medicine. He has also been given the title of "National Famous Physician of Chinese Medicine". As an expert, he has earned national recognition and is assigned as a Master Physician of the National Master and Apprentice Education Program. He was also the former director of the department of Dermatology and STD in Guangdong Provincial Hospital of TCM, consultant for the *Journal of Guangzhou University of Traditional Chinese Medicine*, as well as member of the editorial board for the *New Journal of Traditional Chinese Medicine*. Professor Xuan also serves as a consultant for the following societies: China Association of Chinese Medicine—Dermatology Board, Chinese Association of the Integration of Traditional and Western Medicine—Specialty Board for Dermatology and STD, and Guangdong Association of the Integration of Traditional and Western Medicine—Specialty Board for Dermatology and STD. He is the lifetime director of the Guangdong Provincial Chinese Medicine Association and the honorary director of Guangdong Provincial Specialty Board for Dermatology and External Application of Chinese Medicine. In addition, he is a committee member of Guangdong Provincial and Guangzhou Municipal Special Board for Chinese Medicine.

He has been engaged in clinical practice, teaching, and scientific research for more than 40 years. Over his long career in clinical practice, he has developed the special clinical approach—"tonifying the Kidney"—which is based on the principle of harmonizing yin and yang. The approach has been proved effective in the treatment of complicated dermatological diseases. Naturally, he is widely sought out by patients for treating difficult dermatological cases.

Professor Xuan has published over 60 research papers in several famous Chinese medicine journals, such as *Harmony of Yin and Yang as the Primary Treatment Principle* and *Insights of Clinical Diagnosis and Treatment of Dermatology*. He has edited 5 monographs including *Chinese Medicine Treatment of Dermatology and STD*, *Clinical Diagnosis and Treatment of Dermatology and STD in Chinese Medicine*. He co-authored the widely-used textbook of *Chinese External Medicine*. More recently, he directed 8 research projects at ministry and provincial levels. He has won several clinical and scientific research achievement awards at national and provincial levels.

Foreword

Chinese medicine is a broad and profound art of healing. It is a well-established and comprehensive system of medicine with an ancient origin and a long rich history. Throughout the ages, it has made a significant contribution to the prosperity of the Chinese civilization. The system of pattern differentiation and treatment fully reflects the Chinese medical view of health and disease as a holistic concept, the emphasis on the body's ability to regulate itself and adapt to the environment, and the need for individualized treatment. The integration of diseases and syndromes is the consummation of treatment based on pattern differentiation. It fully displays the superior characteristic of this discipline and has an extensive influence on the development of the art of Chinese medicine.

The intention of this series of books is to introduce accurate Chinese medical diagnosis and treatment of various diseases to overseas readers.

The Chinese edition of *The Clinical Practice of Chinese Medicine* was edited by the Second Teaching Hospital of Guangzhou University of CM (also known as Guangdong Provincial Hospital of TCM), and published by the People's Medical Publishing House. When the series was published in 2000, it was widely accepted in clinical practice due to its originality, distinguishing features, richness in content, completeness, accuracy, and outstanding emphases. This series has become a trademark of standard in the eyes of Chinese and integrative medical practitioners. During the second printing of this series of books, Professor Deng Tie-tao praised, "For a series to be printed a multiple number of times shows that it is highly regarded and has received excellent reviews." In order to keep up with the constant development of medical science, this series was revised and re-published in 2004 by the People's Medical Publishing

House. Due to its popularity, it has been reprinted numerous times since.

The English edition of this series of books includes 20 volumes:

- COPD & Asthma
- Coronary Artery Disease & Hyperlipidemia
- Stroke & Parkinson's Disease
- Chronic Gastritis & Irritable Bowel Syndrome
- Diabetes & Obesity
- Gout & Rheumatoid Arthritis
- Menstrual Disorders I: Dysfunctional Uterine Bleeding & Amenorrhea
- Menstrual Disorders II: Premenstrual Syndrome, Dysmenorrhea & Perimenopause
- Endometriosis & Uterine Fibroids
- Pelvic Inflammatory Disease & Miscarriage
- Postpartum Hypogalactia & Breast Hyperplasia
- Male & Female Infertility
- Urticaria
- Eczema & Atopic Dermatitis
- Lupus Erythematosus
- Scleroderma & Dermatomyositis
- *Acne & Alopecia*
- Psoriasis & Cutaneous Pruritis
- Herpes Zoster & Fungal Skin Infections
- Chloasma & Vitiligo

Clinical application varies by individual and by location; when this is combined with the rapid development of medical science, the treatment methods and medicinal dosages may also vary accordingly. When using these books as a reference guide, overseas readers should confirm the formulas and dosages of medicinals according to the individual health condition of the patient and take into account the origin of the Chinese medicinals.

The quotes in these books were taken from various medical literature during the compilation process. We have deleted some of the contents of the original texts for the purpose of uniformity and ease of reading. We ask for the reader's forgiveness and express our respect and gratitude toward the original authors.

Due to the complicated nature of the diagnoses and treatments covered in these books and the wide range of topics they touch upon, it is inevitable that one may encounter errors while reading through them. We respectfully welcome constructive criticism and corrections from our readers.

The clinical practice of medicine changes with the constant development of medical science. The books in this series will be revised regularly to continuously adapt to the development of traditional Chinese medicine.

Editorial Board for the English edition of
The Clinical Practice of Chinese Medicine **series**

Editorial Board

for the English edition of

The Clinical Practice of Chinese Medicine Series

ACADEMIC CONSULTANTS

Deng Tie-tao

Master of the National Master and Apprentice Education Program, Tenured Professor of Guangzhou University of CM, Former vice President of Guangzhou University of CM

Ren Ji-xue

Master of the National Master and Apprentice Education Program, Professor of Changchun University of CM, Visiting Professor of Guangzhou University of CM

Yan De-xin

Professor of Chinese Medicine, Medical College, Shanghai Railway University, Specialized in the theory & clinical practice of Chinese medicine

Jiao Shu-de

Master of the National Master and Apprentice Education Program, Professor of Chinese Medicine, China-Japan Hospital, Ministry of Health

Lu Zhi-zheng

Master of the National Master and Apprentice Education Program, Professor of Chinese Medicine, China Academy of Chinese Medical Science

Gan Zu-wang

Master of the National Master and Apprentice Education Program, Professor of Chinese Medicine, Nanjing University of TCM, A founder of otolaryngology of Chinese medicine

Wu Xian-zhong
Specialist of Integrative Medicine, Academician of Chinese Academy of Engineering, Professor, Tianjin Medical University, Chairman of Tianjin Institute of Acute Abdomen Research on Integrative Medicine

Chen Ke-ji
Specialist of Cardiovascular & Aging Diseases, Academician of Chinese Academy of Science, Professor of Medicine, Xiyuan Hospital, and Institute of Aging Medicine, China Academy of Chinese Medical Science, Consultant on Traditional Medicine, WHO

Wang Yong-yan
Specialist of Chinese Internal Medicine, Academician of Chinese Academy of Engineering, Professor and former President of Beijing University of CM, and Honorary President of China Academy of Chinese Medical Science

General Coordinator

Lü Yu-bo
Professor & Vice President, Guangzhou University of CM, President, the Second Teaching Hospital of Guangzhou University of CM

Editors-in-Chief

Luo Yun-jian
Guangdong Province Entitled Famous Chinese Medicine Physician, Professor of Chinese Internal Medicine, & former Vice President of the Second Teaching Hospital of Guangzhou University of CM

Liu Mao-cai
Guangdong Province Entitled Famous Chinese Medicine Physician, Professor of Chinese Internal Medicine, & former Vice President of the Second Teaching Hospital of Guangzhou University of CM, Former Chairman of Institute for Aging Cerebral Diseases, Guangzhou University of CM

Associate Editors-in-Chief

Xuan Guo-wei
Guangdong Province Entitled Famous Chinese Medicine Physician, Director & Professor, Department of Chinese External Medicine, Guangzhou University of CM, Former Vice President of the Second Teaching Hospital of Guangzhou University of CM

Huang Chun-lin
Professor of Chinese Internal Medicine, & former Associate-Director of the Second Institute for Clinical Research, Guangzhou University of CM

Chen Da-can
Professor of Chinese External Medicine, Vice President of the Second Teaching Hospital of Guangzhou University of CM

Chen Zhi-qiang
Professor of Chinese External Medicine, Director of the Department of Surgery, Vice President of the Second Teaching Hospital of Guangzhou University of CM

Feng Wei-bin
Professor of Chinese Internal Medicine, the Second Teaching Hospital of Guangzhou University of CM

Yang Zhi-min
Professor of Chinese Internal Medicine, Vice President of the Second Teaching Hospital of Guangzhou University of CM

Lu Chuan-jian
Professor of Chinese External Medicine, Vice President of the Second Teaching Hospital of Guangzhou University of CM

Zou Xu
Professor of Chinese Internal Medicine, Vice President of the Second Teaching Hospital of Guangzhou University of CM

Members (Listed alphabetically by name)

Deng Zhao-zhi

Professor of Chinese Internal Medicine, Guangzhou University of CM

Fan Guan-jie

Professor of Chinese Internal Medicine, Director of Department of Education, the Second Teaching Hospital of Guangzhou University of CM

Fan Rui-qiang

Professor of Chinese External Medicine, Director of Department of Dermatology, the Second Teaching Hospital of Guangzhou University of CM

Huang Jian-ling

Professor of Chinese Medicine Gynecology, Director of the First Department of Gynecology, the Second Teaching Hospital of Guangzhou University of CM

Huang Pei-xin

Professor of Chinese Internal Medicine, the Second Teaching Hospital of Guangzhou University of CM, Head of the Research Project of Cerebral Disease Treatment on Chinese Internal Medicine, Sponsored by SATCM China

Huang Sui-ping

Professor of Chinese Internal Medicine, Director of Department of Digestion, the Second Teaching Hospital of Guangzhou University of CM

Li Li-yun

Guangdong Province Entitled Famous Chinese Medicine Physician, Professor of Chinese Medicine Gynecology, the Second Teaching Hospital of Guangzhou University of CM

Liang Xue-fang

Professor of Chinese Medicine Gynecology, Director of the Third Department of Gynecology, the Second Teaching Hospital of Guangzhou University of CM

Lin Lin

Professor of Chinese Internal Medicine, Director of Department of Respiratory, the Second Teaching Hospital of Guangzhou University of CM

Liu Wei-sheng

Master of the National Master and Apprentice Education Program, Professor of Chinese Internal Medicine, the Second Teaching Hospital of Guangzhou University of CM

Wang Xiao-yun

Professor of Chinese Medicine Gynecology, Director of Department of Gynecology, Head of Teaching Division of Gynecology, the Second Teaching Hospital of Guangzhou University of CM

Lin Yi

Professor of Mastopathy in Chinese Medicine, the Second Teaching Hospital of Guangzhou University of CM, Head of the National Key Subject –Mastopathy in Chinese Medicine

Si-tu Yi

Professor of Chinese Medicine Gynecology, the Second Teaching Hospital of Guangzhou University of CM, Head of the National Key Subject – Chinese Medicine Gynecology

SPONSORED BY

The Second Teaching Hospital of Guangzhou University of CM, also known as **Guangdong Provincial Hospital of TCM**

Preface

This publication is an important component text in the series *The Clinical Practice of Chinese Medicine*. The intention of this book is to introduce the Chinese medical experience to our overseas readers, while also offering the latest developments in Chinese medical dermatology. The rich and valuable content in this book is rooted in the accumulated knowledge of several thousand of years of documented clinical experience. At the same time, recent progress has been made in the clinical treatment of difficult diseases like eczema, psoriasis, vitiligo, and hair loss using modern integrative approaches.

Acne, alopecia areata and androgenetic alopecia are three diseases most commonly seen in the dermatology clinic. Because acne primarily affects the face, many individuals feel self-conscious and actively seek out treatments to improve their appearance. Fortunately, the treatment of acne with Chinese medicine has progressed significantly in the last ten years. The standard etiologies of acne have now expanded beyond the traditional categories of wind heat, lung heat, and blood heat to also include patterns of damp-heat, blood stasis, phlegm bind, insufficient kidney yin, and hyperactivity of the ministerial fire. These new perspectives have given new direction and meaning to the clinical treatment of acne and other tenacious skin conditions.

Alopecia areata is another commonly encountered dermatological disease. Its pathogenesis and associated syndromes are also examined in great depth. In recent years, people have become significantly affected by fast-paced lifestyles, increasing work pressures, and environmental pollution, all of which stress the immune system. Alopecia areata is currently categorized into three major Chinese medicine patterns: kidney deficiency, blood deficiency, and blood stasis.

Androgenetic alopecia is another common form of hair loss that occurs in both men and women. In the early stage, it is generally associated with blood-heat, wind dryness, and spleen-stomach damp-heat; while in the late stage, liver and kidney deficiency is generally involved. According to the presenting signs and symptoms, Chinese medicinals may be applied to cool the blood, eliminate wind, fortify the spleen, dispel dampness, and nourish the liver and kidney.

The authors of this text are Chinese medical doctors who specialize in dermatology. They have accumulated a great deal of experience through their years of clinical practice, and are also the authors of many dermatology textbooks. This book provides a detailed introduction to TCM syndrome differentiation as applied to the clinical treatment of dermatological diseases. It also features comprehensive theoretical discussions and current perspectives on the major points and challenges of this subject.

In this series, readers will find an organized and thorough presentation of each disease which includes: a brief overview, etiology and pathomechanism, Chinese medical treatment, prognosis, preventative healthcare, case studies, experience of renowned physicians, integrative treatment approaches, quotes from classical texts, and modern research. The **brief overview** offers a general introduction to the biomedical view of each disease. The **Chinese medical etiology**, **pathomechanism**, and **Chinese medical treatment** sections represent the central focus and foundation of the book. **Preventative healthcare**, **case studies**, and **integrative treatment approaches** present more current perspectives and also many unique methods of treatment. **Quotes from classical texts and modern research** provide even further resources for study.

This series presents a clear description of each disease and also the key points for diagnosis and treatment using Chinese medicine. Further detail is provided by presenting the clinical experiences of both ancient and modern-day renowned physicians.

In order to ensure a better understanding of the contents of this Chinese medical book series, we have recognized that different readers have different needs and desires.

First, both medical professionals and students can read this series for professional study and application. To fully appreciate this work, a solid background in the basic theory of Chinese medicine and an understanding of the classical formulas is required. The reader should also be familiar with the properties of each individual medicinal as well as their contraindications, incompatibilities, and proper dosages.

Second, readers who are more generally interested in Chinese medicine should pay attention to the characteristics, advantages, and special methods of Chinese medicine with regards to preventative healthcare. Chinese medicinals should be prescribed only under the guidance of professional Chinese medical physicians.

We hope that these books will become useful and valuable to everyone in the field of Chinese medicine, as well as for biomedical physicians with an interest in Chinese medicine. Hopefully, this book can help the reader gain a deeper understanding of Chinese medical diagnosis and treatment, particularly in the field of dermatology. Through the discussion of integrative treatment approaches, we also aim to bridge the gap between traditional Chinese medicine and current biomedical practices.

Due to the rapidly advancing nature of clinical medicine, we apologize for any out-dated or incorrect information that may appear in these books. We hope that our readers will not hesitate to offer their comments and suggestions on how to improve the content of this material.

Fan Rui-qiang & Xuan Guo-wei

April 2008

Contents

Acne ... 1

OVERVIEW ... 5
CHINESE MEDICAL ETIOLOGY AND PATHOMECHANISM ... 6
CHINESE MEDICAL TREATMENT ... 9
    Pattern Differentiation and Treatment ... 9
    Additional Treatment Modalities ... 14
PROGNOSIS ... 18
PREVENTIVE HEALTHCARE ... 19
    Lifestyle Modification ... 19
    Dietary Recommendation ... 19
    Regulation of Emotional and Mental Health ... 20
CLINICAL EXPERIENCE OF RENOWNED PHYSICIANS ... 21
    Empirical Formulas ... 21
    Selected Case Studies ... 23
    Discussions ... 28
PERSPECTIVES OF INTEGRATIVE MEDICINE ... 32
    Challenges and Solutions ... 32
    Insight from Empirical Wisdom ... 34
    Summary ... 36
SELECTED QUOTES FROM CLASSICAL TEXTS ... 38
MODERN RESEARCH ... 39
    Clinical Research ... 39
    Experimental Studies ... 63
REFERENCES ... 67

Alopecia Areata — 71

OVERVIEW	75
CHINESE MEDICAL ETIOLOGY AND PATHOMECHANISM	77
CHINESE MEDICAL TREATMENT	77
Pattern Differentiation and Treatment	77
Additional Treatment Modalities	86
PROGNOSIS	94
PREVENTIVE HEALTHCARE	95
Regulation of Emotional and Mental Health	95
Lifestyle Modification	95
Dietary Recommendation	96
CLINICAL EXPERIENCE OF RENOWNED PHYSICIANS	99
Empirical Formulas	99
Selected Case Studies	103
Discussions	108
PERSPECTIVES OF INTEGRATIVE MEDICINE	114
Challenges and Solutions	114
Insight from Empirical Wisdom	117
Summary	122
SELECTED QUOTES FROM CLASSICAL TEXTS	131
MODERN RESEARCH	136
Clinical Research	136
Experimental Studies	148
REFERENCES	151

Androgenetic Alopecia ... 155

- **OVERVIEW** ... 159
- **CHINESE MEDICAL ETIOLOGY AND PATHOMECHANISM** ... 161
- **CHINESE MEDICAL TREATMENT** ... 161
  - Pattern Differentiation and Treatment ... 162
  - Additional Treatment Modalities ... 167
- **PROGNOSIS** ... 174
- **PREVENTIVE HEALTHCARE** ... 174
  - Lifestyle Modification ... 174
  - Dietary Recommendation ... 175
  - Regulation of Emotional and Mental Health ... 178
- **CLINICAL EXPERIENCE OF RENOWNED PHYSICIANS** ... 178
  - Empirical Formulas ... 178
  - Selected Case Studies ... 182
  - Discussions ... 192
- **PERSPECTIVES OF INTEGRATIVE MEDICINE** ... 200
  - Challenges and Solutions ... 200
  - Insight from Empirical Wisdom ... 202
  - Summary ... 206
- **SELECTED QUOTES FROM CLASSICAL TEXTS** ... 206
- **MODERN RESEARCH** ... 208
  - Clinical Research ... 208
  - Experimental Studies ... 220
- **REFERENCES** ... 225

Index by Disease Names and Symptoms ... 229
Index by Chinese Medicinals and Formulas ... 232
General Index ... 239

Acne

by

Fan Rui-qiang
Chief Physician & Professor of Chinese External Medicine

Huang Yong-jing, M.S. TCM
Associate Chief Physician of Chinese External Medicine

Xuan Guo-wei
Chief Physician & Professor of Chinese External Medicine

Wu Wei, M.S. TCM
Attending Physician of Chinese External Medicine

002 Acne & Alopecia

OVERVIEW ... 5
CHINESE MEDICAL ETIOLOGY AND PATHOMECHANISM ... 6
CHINESE MEDICAL TREATMENT ... 9
Pattern Differentiation and Treatment ... 9
Additional Treatment Modalities ... 14
1. Chinese Patent Medicine ... 14
2. Acupuncture and Moxibustion ... 15
3. External Application ... 16
4. Clearing Acne ... 17
5. Chinese Medicinal Facial Mask ... 17
6. Simple Prescriptions and Empirical Formulas ... 17

PROGNOSIS ... 18
PREVENTIVE HEALTHCARE ... 19
Lifestyle Modification ... 19
Dietary Recommendation ... 19
Regulation of Emotional and Mental Health ... 20

CLINICAL EXPERIENCE OF RENOWNED PHYSICIANS ... 21
Empirical Formulas ... 21
1. Modified Pí Pá Qīng Fèi Yǐn (枇杷清肺饮) (Zhu Ren-kang) ... 21
2. Cuò Chuāng Píng (痤疮平) (Xu Yi-hou) ... 22
3. Píng Cuò Tāng (平痤汤) (Lu De-ming) ... 23

Selected Case Studies ... 23
1. Case Studies of Zhu Ren-kang: Cystic Acne ... 23
2. Case Studies of Lu De-ming: Lung Heat Damaging Yin ... 25
3. Case Studies of Guan Fen: Lung and Stomach Heat ... 27

Discussions ... 28
1. Zhu Ren-kang on the Two Types of Acne ... 28
2. Lu De-ming on Hyperactivity of Fire due to Yin Deficiency ... 29
3. Xu Yi-hou on "Four Differentiations" and "Ten Treatments" for Acne ... 31

PERSPECTIVES OF INTEGRATIVE MEDICINE ... 32

Challenges and Solutions ... 32
Challenge #1: How to Prevent Recurrence ... 33
Challenge #2: How to Treat Severe Acne ... 33
Insight from Empirical Wisdom ... 34
1. Treating Acne from the Kidney ... 34
2. Dān Shēn (Radix et Rhizoma Salviae Miltiorrhizae) and Acne Treatment ... 35
3. Perspectives of Integrative Medicine ... 36
Summary ... 36
SELECTED QUOTES FROM CLASSICAL TEXTS ... 38
MODERN RESEARCH ... 39
Clinical Research ... 39
1. Pattern Differentiation and Corresponding Treatment ... 39
2. Treatment ... 39
Experimental Studies ... 63
1. Research on The Efficacy of Single Chinese Medicinals ... 63
2. Research on Bacteriostatic Chinese Medicinal Formulas ... 64
3. Research on Chinese Medicinals and Sebum Secretion ... 66
4. Dān Shēn (Radix et Rhizoma Salviae Miltiorrhizae) Acne Treatment ... 67
REFERENCES ... 67

OVERVIEW

Acne is a chronic dermatological disease of the sebaceous glands and follicles associated with endocrine dysfunction. Acne often affects teenagers, appearing particularly on the face with repeated occurrences. The clinical features of acne include the appearance of papules, pustules, nodules, and cysts. Acne is a very common disease. According to Chinese medical literature, acne occurs in 20%-24% of the general population and even at higher rates among individuals in puberty, reaching 30%-50%. Medical statistics in some regions outside of China have indicated that acne can occur in up to 90% of their populations. Acne typically affects men more than women; however, women are more apt to seek treatments due to aesthetic and cosmetic reasons. Because acne primarily affects the face, people tend to be more self-conscious, leading them to seek out more effective methods of prevention and treatment, especially with today's higher standard of living.

In biomedicine, acne is seen as a skin disease with multiple causes. Primary causes include high androgenic hormone levels in the blood serum or skin tissue, excessive sebaceous gland secretions, follicular hyperkeratosis, and local bacterial infection. Moreover, acne is also thought to be related to various factors such as immune reactions, genetics, and hemorheology. High androgenic hormones due to endocrine imbalances can result in excessive sebaceous gland secretions. Excessive sebum secretions can cause keratosis and hyperplasia of hair follicles and sebaceous gland ducts, thereby blocking the sebaceous glands and inhibiting sebum excretion, which can lead to the appearance of acne and papules. At puberty, acne often occurs on the forehead, cheeks, chin and periphery of the mouth, or even on the chest, back, and upper arms. Initially, it appears as small blackheads or whiteheads with a cutaneous fatty secretion that can be squeezed out. In some cases, small red papules may appear at the initial stage. Later, it develops into small pustules and nodules. In severe cases, the condition may present with painful abscesses, cysts, or inflammation of cellular tissue. With excessive sebaceous gland secretions, other symptoms will emerge such as red, oily and itchy skin. If acne continues to recur, the skin will display uneven scar tissue and hyperpigmentation. Based on the appearance and its pathogenic condition, acne can be divided into seven types: acne papules, acne pustules, acne nodules, acne cysts, acne conglobata, atrophic acne and acne cachecticorum.

In clinic, we should first inspect for mites and ticks, pityrosporion ovale (an organism responsible for dandruff), and bacteria in order to rule out other skin conditions and to formulate an accurate diagnosis. There are three treatment approaches in biomedicine:

(1) Inhibit excessive sebaceous gland secretion.

(2) Reduce keratosis and hyperplasia of the follicles and sebaceous gland ducts.

(3) Eliminate bacteria and inflammation of the follicle.

Main treatments include the administration of antibiotics, retinol, estrogen, corticosteroids, vitamins, and other androgen antagonists. In severe cases, different medications are prescribed in combination. Antibiotic medications for acne include tetracycline, minocycline, roxithromycin, clindamycin, and erythromycin. Other treatments include local injections at the affected area, cryotherapy, and photon therapy. All of these treatments may improve the condition to some degree.

In Chinese medicine, the disease name is referred to as "lung wind acne".

CHINESE MEDICAL ETIOLOGY AND PATHOMECHANISM

In Chinese medicine, "lung wind acne" is caused by congenital insufficiency of kidney yin, and hyperactivity of the ministerial fire and *tian gui*. Additionally, an unhealthy diet and lifestyle may lead to lung and stomach fire steaming the face, which then leads to blood heat and blood stasis.

(1) Kidney Yin Deficiency

The kidney is the root of the congenital constitution. It stores essence and governs reproduction, growth and development. *Tian gui* from the kidney directly impacts physical growth, development, and reproduction. For instance, *Plain Questions–Treatise of Heavenly Truth From Remote Antiquity* (*Sù Wèn–Shàng Gǔ Tiān Zhēn Lùn*, 素问·上古天真论) states:

"For females, when they are seven, they have sufficient kidney qi, new teeth grow in, and the hair is growing. When they are fourteen, *tian gui* begins to take effect, the penetrating vessel is flourishing, and menarche arrives, so they can procreate;… when they are forty nine, the conception vessel is insufficient, the penetrating vessel declines, *tian gui* becomes exhausted, menostasia appears, causing a poor appearance and an inability to procreate. For males, when they are eight, they have sufficient kidney qi, growing hair, and new teeth; when they are sixteen, they have flourishing kidney qi, *tian gui* begins to take effect, essential qi is overflowing, and yin-yang is in harmony, so they can procreate;… when they are fifty eight, liver qi declines, the sinews are unable to move, *tian gui* becomes exhausted, essential qi is lacking, kidney declines, and the physique and body are poor…"(女子七岁，肾气盛，齿更，发长；二七而天癸至，任脉通，太冲脉盛，月事以时下，故有子；……七七任脉虚，太冲脉衰少，天癸竭，地道不通，故形坏而无子也。丈夫八岁，肾气实，发长齿更；二八，肾气盛，天癸至，精气溢泻，阴阳和，故能有子；……七八，肝气衰，筋不能动，天癸竭，精少，肾脏衰，形体皆极……)

Constitutional kidney yin deficiency leads to disharmony of kidney yin and yang. When girls are about fourteen and boys are about sixteen, it causes hyperactivity of the ministerial fire and *tian gui*. As a result, these young individuals grow and develop too early, and this may develop into acne. So, the main causes of lung wind acne are insufficient kidney yin leading to kidney yin and yang disharmony, and hyperactivity of the ministerial fire and *tian gui*.

(2) Blood Heat in the Lung and Stomach Channels

The face is primarily governed by the lung and stomach channels. *Plain Questions–Generation of Five Organs* (*Sù Wèn–Wǔ Zàng Shēng Chéng Piān* 素问·五脏生成篇) states: "The lung is connected with the skin, and hair is its mirror." (肺之合皮也，其荣毛也。)

In the theory of five phases, the lung belongs to metal and the kidney belongs to water. With constitutional kidney yin deficiency, yin cannot rise to enrich the lung, which leads to lung yin deficiency. In addition, the lung and the large intestine are interior-exterior related organs. With the overeating of fatty meats, refined grains, and rich foods too difficult to digest, the large intestine will accumulate heat that steams the lung and stomach. All of the above scenarios will result in blood heat in the lung and stomach channels, thereby creating facial acne, papules, and pustules.

(3) Phlegm and Blood Stasis Binding Together

Prolonged kidney yin deficiency or blood heat in lung and stomach channels scorches body fluids, creating phlegm. Yin deficiency leads to the inhibited flow of blood, resulting in blood stasis. Phlegm and blood stasis binding together on the face will manifest with nodules, cysts, and scarring.

(4) Disharmony of the Penetrating and Conception Vessels

If kidney yin is deficient and the liver fails to circulate qi properly, there will be disharmony in the penetrating and conception vessels. The penetrating vessel is the sea of blood and the conception vessel governs the uterus and pregnancy. If these two channels have disharmonies, the sea of blood cannot be nourished in time, menstruation will be irregular, and facial acne will worsen before or after menstruation.

CHINESE MEDICAL TREATMENT

Based on the etiology and pathomechanism of acne, the primary treatment principle of Chinese medicine is to enrich yin and drain fire, clear the lung and resolve toxins, cool and invigorate the blood, and regulate the penetrating and conception vessels. For beneficial results, internal and external treatment should be combined to treat the root and branch simultaneously. Chinese medicine should be combined with biomedicine for the treatment of more severe cases.

Pattern Differentiation and Treatment

According to its duration and appearance, acne is generally differentiated into three patterns for treatment: yin deficiency generating internal heat, static heat and phlegm binding together, and disharmony of the penetrating and conception vessels. Among them, yin deficiency generating internal heat is the basic pattern which could further develop into the other two patterns.

(1) Yin Deficiency Generating Internal Heat

【Syndrome Characteristics】

Red facial pimples, or with pustules and nodules. Dry mouth, vexation, insomnia and dream-disturbed sleep, dry and hard stools, and short voidings of reddish urine. Red tongue with thin and yellowish coating, and a rapid or rapid thready pulse.

【Treatment Principle】

To nourish yin, drain fire, clear the lung, and cool the blood.

【Commonly Used Medicinals】

Use *dān shēn* (Radix et Rhizoma Salviae Miltiorrhizae), *nǚ zhēn zǐ* (Fructus Ligustri Lucidi), *hàn lián cǎo* (Herba Ecliptae), *shēng dì* (Radix Rehmanniae), *zhī mǔ* (Rhizoma Anemarrhenae), and *zé xiè* (Rhizoma Alismatis) to nourish yin and drain fire.

【Representative Formula】

Xiāo Cuò Tāng (消痤汤).

【Ingredients】

女贞子	nǚ zhēn zǐ	20g	Fructus Ligustri Lucidi
旱莲草	hàn lián cǎo	20g	Herba Ecliptae
知母	zhī mǔ	12g	Rhizoma Anemarrhenae
黄柏	huáng bǎi	12g	Cortex Phellodendri Chinensis
鱼腥草	yú xīng cǎo	20g	Herba Houttuyniae
蒲公英	pú gōng yīng	15g	Herba Taraxaci
连翘	lián qiào	15g	Fructus Forsythiae
生地黄	shēng dì huáng	15g	Radix Rehmanniae
丹参	dān shēn	25g	Radix et Rhizoma Salviae Miltiorrhizae
甘草	gān cǎo	3g	Radix et Rhizoma Glycyrrhizae

One bag per day. Decoct in 500 ml of water until 200 ml remains. Drink warm.

【Formula Analysis】

Nǚ zhēn zǐ (Fructus Ligustri Lucidi) and *hàn lián cǎo* (Herba Ecliptae) nourish the kidney yin while *zhī mǔ* (Rhizoma Anemarrhenae) and *huáng bǎi* (Cortex Phellodendri Chinensis) drain kidney fire. In the two groups of medicinals, one is to nourish and the other is to drain, so together they regulate and balance kidney yin and yang. *Yú xīng cǎo* (Herba Houttuyniae), *pú gōng yīng* (Herba Taraxaci), *lián qiào* (Fructus Forsythiae) clear heat, diffuse the lung, resolve toxins, and reduce swelling. *Shēng dì huáng* (Radix Rehmanniae) and *dān shēn* (Radix et Rhizoma Salviae Miltiorrhizae) clear heat, cool blood, and invigorate the blood to transform stasis. *Gān cǎo* (Radix et Rhizoma Glycyrrhizae) resolves toxins, clears heat, and harmonizes the actions of other medicinals.

【Modifications】

➤ For constipation with hard stools, add *dà huáng* (Radix et Rhizoma Rhei) 10g (decoct later) and *zhǐ shí* (Fructus Aurantii Immaturus) 12g to clear heat and free the bowels.

➤ For loose watery stools with a thick greasy tongue coating, remove *shēng dì huáng* (Radix Rehmanniae) and add *tǔ fú líng* (Rhizoma Smilacis Glabrae) 15g and *yīn chén hāo* (Artemisiae Scopariae) 20g to drain dampness, clear heat and resolve toxins.

➤ For insomnia and dream-disturbed sleep, add *hé huān pí* (Cortex Albiziae) 15g and *fú líng* (Poria) 20g to calm the heart and quiet the spirit.

➤ For exuberant lung-stomach heat, add *shēng shí gāo* (raw Gypsum Fibrosum) 20g and *dì gǔ pí* (Cortex Lycii) 15g to clear and drain lung-stomach fire.

(2) Static Heat and Phlegm Binding Together

【Pattern Characteristics】

Red or dark red facial nodules, cysts, and scarred depressions associated with small pustules, acne and hyperpigmentation. Red or dark red tongue with stasis spots, and a thin yellowish coating. The pulse is wiry and slippery, or thready and choppy.

【Treatment Principle】

To nourish yin and clear heat, transform stasis and dissipate nodules.

【Commonly Used Medicinals】

Use *dāng guī* (Radix Angelicae Sinensis), *hóng huā* (Flos Carthami), *táo rén* (Semen Persicae), *chì sháo* (Radix Paeoniae Rubra), *yù jīn* (Radix Curcumae), and *dān shēn* (Radix et Rhizoma Salviae Miltiorrhizae) to transform stasis and dissipate nodules.

【Representative Formula】

Modifications of *Táo Hóng Sì Wù Tāng* (桃红四物汤) and *Xiāo Cuò*

Tāng (消痤汤).

【Ingredients】

生地黄	shēng dì huáng	15g	Radix Rehmanniae
红花	hóng huā	6g	Flos Carthami
赤芍	chì sháo	10g	Radix Paeoniae Rubra
丹参	dān shēn	30g	Radix et Rhizoma Salviae Miltiorrhizae
女贞子	nǔ zhēn zǐ	20g	Fructus Ligustri Lucidi
旱莲草	hàn lián cǎo	20g	Herba Ecliptae
鱼腥草	yú xīng cǎo	15g	Herba Houttuyniae
蒲公英	pú gōng yīng	15g	Herba Taraxaci
郁金	yù jīn	10g	Radix Curcumae
甘草	gān cǎo	3g	Radix et Rhizoma Glycyrrhizae

One bag per day. Decoct in 500 ml of water until 200 ml remains. Drink warm.

【Formula Analysis】

Shēng dì huáng (Radix Rehmanniae), nǔ zhēn zǐ (Fructus Ligustri Lucidi), hàn lián cǎo (Herba Ecliptae) nourish yin and clear heat. Dān shēn (Radix et Rhizoma Salviae Miltiorrhizae), hóng huā (Flos Carthami), and yù jīn (Radix Curcumae) transform stasis, disperse phlegm and dissipate nodules. Yú xīng cǎo (Herba Houttuyniae) and pú gōng yīng (Herba Taraxaci) clear heat and diffuse the lung, resolve toxins, and reduce swelling. Gān cǎo (Radix et Rhizoma Glycyrrhizae) resolves toxins, clears heat, and harmonizes the actions of other medicinals.

【Modifications】

➢ For cysts with bloody pus, add zào jiǎo cì (Spina Gleditsiae) 12g, chuān shān jiǎ (Squama Manis) 10g (decoct first), and bái zhǐ (Radix Angelicae Dahuricae) 10g to reduce swelling and expel pus.

➢ For severe painful nodules, add xuán shēn (Radix Scrophulariae) 20g and zhè bèi mǔ (Bulbus Fritillariae Thunbergii) 12g to clear heat, resolve toxins, and dissipate nodules.

> For scarring, increase *dān shēn* (Radix et Rhizoma Salviae Miltiorrhizae) to 50g to increase the effect of invigorating blood and transforming stasis.

(3) Disharmony of the Penetrating and Conception Vessels

【Pattern Characteristics】

In females, the occurrence and severity of acne are closely connected to the menstrual cycle. Before menstruation, more facial acne can appear with greater severity. After menstruation, the condition may improve. There may be irregular menstruation with vexation, irritability, and distending pain in the breasts before menstruation. Red tongue with thin and yellowish coating, and a wiry, thready and rapid pulse.

【Treatment Principle】

Nourish yin and clear heat, regulate the penetrating and conception vessels.

【Commonly Used Medicinals】

Use *chái hú* (Radix Bupleuri), *yù jīn* (Radix Curcumae), *nǚ zhēn zǐ* (Fructus Ligustri Lucidi), *hàn lián cǎo* (Herba Ecliptae), *pú gōng yīng* (Herba Taraxaci), and *shān zhā* (Fructus Crataegi) to regulate the penetrating and conception vessels.

【Representative Formula】

Modifications of *Chái Hú Shū Gān Tāng* (柴胡疏肝汤) and *Xiāo Cuò Tāng* (消痤汤).

【Ingredients】

柴胡	chái hú	10g	Radix Bupleuri
郁金	yù jīn	15g	Radix Curcumae
白芍	bái sháo	15g	Radix Paeoniae Alba
女贞子	nǚ zhēn zǐ	20g	Fructus Ligustri Lucidi
旱莲草	hàn lián cǎo	20g	Herba Ecliptae
鱼腥草	yú xīng cǎo	15g	Herba Houttuyniae
蒲公英	pú gōng yīng	15g	Herba Taraxaci

丹参	dān shēn	15g	Radix et Rhizoma Salviae Miltiorrhizae
山楂	shān zhā	15g	Fructus Crataegi
甘草	gān cǎo	3g	Radix et Rhizoma Glycyrrhizae

One bag per day. Decoct in 500 ml of water until 200 ml remains. Drink warm.

【Formula Analysis】

Chái hú (Radix Bupleuri), *yù jīn* (Radix Curcumae), and *bái sháo* (Radix Paeoniae Alba) course the liver, and regulate the penetrating and conception vessels. *Nǔ zhēn zǐ* (Fructus Ligustri Lucidi) and *hàn lián cǎo* (Herba Ecliptae) enrich the kidney, nourish yin, and harmonize *tian gui*. *Yú xīng cǎo* (Herba Houttuyniae) and *pú gōng yīng* (Herba Taraxaci) clear heat and diffuse the lung, resolve toxins, and reduce swelling. *Dān shēn* (Radix et Rhizoma Salviae Miltiorrhizae) cools blood and transforms stasis. *Shān zhā* (Fructus Crataegi) disperses stagnation and transforms stasis. *Gān cǎo* (Radix et Rhizoma Glycyrrhizae) resolves toxins, clears heat, and harmonizes the actions of other medicinals.

【Modifications】

➢ For delayed menstruation, breast distention, and vague pain of the lower abdomen, add *xiāng fù* (Rhizoma Cyperi) 15g and *wáng bù liú xíng* (Semen Vaccariae) 12g to promote menstruation and allieviate pain.

➢ For early menstruation, remove *dān shēn* (Radix et Rhizoma Salviae Miltiorrhizae), and add *yì mǔ cǎo* (Herba Leonuri) 25g and *xiāng fù* (Rhizoma Cyperi) 15g to regulate menstruation and clear heat.

Additional Treatment Modalities

1. Chinese Patent Medicine

(1) *Zhī Bǎi Dì Huáng Wán* (知柏地黄丸)

One bolus, twice a day. Take with warm water. Indicated for yin deficiency and internal heat.

(2) *Méi Huā Diǎn Shé Wán* (梅花点舌丸)

1-2 pills, three times a day. Take with warm water. Indicated for phlegm, stasis and heat binding.

(3) *Dān Zhī Xiāo Yáo Wán* (丹栀逍遥丸)

One bolus, three times a day. Take with warm water. Indicated for liver constraint and qi stagnation, and disharmony of the penetrating and conception vessels.

2. Acupuncture and Moxibustion

(1) Acupuncture

【Point Combination】

ST 7	*xià guān*	下关
ST 6	*jiá chē*	颊车
BL 2	*cuán zhú*	攒竹
ST 36	*zú sān lǐ*	足三里
LI 4	*hé gǔ*	合谷
LI 11	*qū chí*	曲池
SP 6	*sān yīn jiāo*	三阴交

【Manipulation】

Use even supplementation and drainage, and retain needles for 15 minutes. Treat once every two days. Seven treatments constitute one course of treatment.

(2) Bloodletting Therapy

【Point Combination】

ear apex	HX6	*ěr jiān*	耳尖
endocrine	CO18	*nèi fēn mì*	内分泌
subcortex	AT4	*pí zhì xià*	皮质下

【Manipulation】

Perform antiseptic cleaning procedures, and then quickly prick to bleed with a three-edged needle. Treat once every two days. Ten treatments constitute one course of treatment.

(3) Acupuncture Point Ear Seed Pressing

【Point Combination】

lung	CO14	*fèi*	肺
endocrine	CO18	*nèi fēn mì*	内分泌
subcortex	AT4	*pí zhì xià*	皮质下

【Manipulation】

Put *wáng bù liú xíng* (Semen Vaccariae) on the center of a small adhesive fabric, and then adhere it to the ear acupuncture point. The patient should to press the point for ten minutes, several times a day. Ten days constitute one course of treatment.

(4) Auricular Needle-embedding Therapy

【Point Combination】

lung	CO14	*fèi*	肺
stomach	CO4	*wèi*	胃
adrenal gland	TG2p	*shèn shàng xiàn*	肾上腺
endocrine	CO18	*nèi fēn mì*	内分泌
subcortex	AT4	*pí zhì xià*	皮质下

【Manipulation】

After antiseptic procedures, imbed an intradermal needle into the ear point. The patient should press it for ten minutes, several times a day.

3. External Application

(1) Apply *Cuò Líng Dīng* (痤灵酊), on the affected area 2-3 times a day. In the winter, select *Cuò Líng Shuāng* (痤灵霜) instead.

(2) Apply 2% of *Lù Méi Sù Sān Huáng Xǐ Jì* (氯霉素三黄洗剂) on the affected area.

(3) Apply *Jīn Sù Lán Dīng* (金粟兰酊) onto the areas with dusky red

scarring.

(4) Chinese Medicinal Facial Mask

Mix *Xiāo Cuò Sǎn* (消痤散) (or another Chinese medicinal powder) with honey. Apply it on the affected area for 20-30 minutes. Apply this medicinal mask daily or every other day. In cases with inflammation, add bitter melon juice to the mask. For hyperpigmentation cases, add tomato juice.

(5) For severe acne with large red nodules or cysts, apply *Sì Huáng Gāo* (四黄膏) to the affected area.

4. Clearing Acne

When there are many blackheads or whiteheads, antiseptic procedures should be used. Then the affected area can be pricked, extracted and drained.

5. Chinese Medicinal Facial Mask

This method applies Chinese medicinals as an effective external therapy. Wash the face with a facial cleanser, spray a mist over the face with an ionized spray, and massage the face. Then apply a Chinese medicinal mask over the skin lesions. Cover the eyes, nose, mouth, and beard with absorbent cotton. Then mix *shēng shí gāo* powder (raw Gypsum Fibrosum) and water into a pasty mask and apply it to the face. Wait until the mask hardens and begins to cool, then it can be removed. Not recommended for patients with significant inflammation.

6. Simple Prescriptions and Empirical Formulas

(1) Use 1-2 pieces of *bái guǒ* (Semen Ginkgo), and cut into tiny slices. Clean the face and then rub these slices into the affected area. Do this daily before bedtime. The acne will typically heal within 7-14 applications.

(2) Decoct *bái huā shé shé cǎo* (Herba Hedyotis Diffusae) 30g, *dān shēn* (Radix et Rhizoma Salviae Miltiorrhizae) 30g and *gān cǎo* (Radix et Rhizoma Glycyrrhizae) 10g in water. One bag per day. This remedy is appropriate for all types of acne.

(3) *Xǐ Liǎn Měi Róng Tāng* (洗脸美容汤)

猪胆汁	zhū dǎn zhī	2-4ml	pig's bile
鲜桃树叶	xiān táo shù yè	50g	fresh peach leaves
鲜槐树叶	xiān huái shù yè	40g	fresh Chinese scholartree leaves

Decoct the two kinds of leaves in water. Add pig bile to the decoction when warm, and stir. Use this decoction to wash the face twice a day, once each morning and evening.

(4) *Shé Dǎn Shuāng* (蛇胆霜)

Add 5 ml of pallas pit viper bile into 500 ml of common facial cream, and mix evenly. Apply the cream to the affected area twice a day.

(5) *Yuè Shí Sǎn* (月石散)

飞甘石	fēi gān shí	4.5g	Calamina
梅片	méi piàn	4.5g	Borneolum
黄丹	huáng dān	3g	Plumbum rubrum

Grind the above medicinals into an extremely fine powder. Take a little powder and mix it with water in the palm of the hand to create a paste. Apply to the affected area before bedtime. Wash off the paste the next morning.

PROGNOSIS

After acne has healed, the symptoms will obviously improve. However, shortly after treatment, secondary hyperpigmentation may appear. Within 3 to 6 months, this condition fades gradually and the skin becomes normal in appearance. However, when severe cases of facial acne are not properly treated, secondary scarring, pimples, or permanent hyperpigmentation can appear.

PREVENTIVE HEALTHCARE

Lifestyle Modification

(1) Avoid eating spicy and fried foods. Eat more fresh fruits and vegetables.

(2) Maintain regular bowel movements.

(3) Do not squeeze acne pimples with the fingers, and use acne medicine cautiously.

(4) If lung wind acne is associated with menstruation, treatment should begin a week before the period begins.

(5) When excessive sebum gives the face an oily and greasy appearance, the face should be washed more often.

Dietary Recommendation

(1) *Kūn Bù Hǎi Zǎo Shòu Ròu Tāng* (昆布海藻瘦肉汤)

昆布	kūn bù	30g	Thallus Laminariae
海藻	hǎi zǎo	30g	Sargassum
红枣	hóng zǎo	5g	Fructus Jujubae
猪瘦肉		500g	lean pork

Clean the herbs and soak them for a few minutes. Remove the pit from the *hóng zǎo* (Fructus Jujubae) and cut the pork into small pieces. Then put all ingredients into a cooking pot, add water, and decoct for about 2 hours over low heat. This remedy is appropriate for acne associated with phlegm, heat and stasis binding.

(2) *Sāng Xìng Zhū Fèi Tāng* (桑杏猪肺汤)

| 桑叶 | sāng yè | 30g | Folium Mori |

| 北杏仁 | běi xìng rén | 10g | Semen Armeniacae Amarum |
| 猪肺 | | 500g | pig lung |

Rinse the herbs and soak them for a few minutes in water. Clean the pig lung and cut it into pieces. Place all ingredients into a cooking pot, add some water, and cook for about 2 hours over low heat. This remedy is appropriate for acne associated with wind heat in the lung channel.

(3) Shēng Mài Bǎi Hé Shòu Ròu Tāng (生麦百合瘦肉汤)

生地	shēng dì	30g	Radix Rehmanniae
麦冬	mài dōng	15g	Radix Ophiopogonis
百合	bǎi hé	30g	Bulbus Lilii
猪瘦肉		500g	lean pork

Clean the herbs and soak them for a few minutes in water. Clean the pork and cut it into pieces. Put all ingredients into a cooking pot, add some water, and cook for about 2 hours over low heat. This remedy is appropriate for acne associated with yin deficiency generating internal heat.

(4) Yáng Shēn Shòu Ròu Tāng (洋参瘦肉汤)

西洋参	xī yáng shēn	20g	Radix Panacis Quinquefolii
蜜枣	mì zǎo	2	preserved jujube date
猪瘦肉		500g	lean pork

Soak the contents in water and bring to a boil. Then decoct over low heat for 2-3 hours. This remedy is appropriate for acne associated with yin deficiency generating internal heat and disharmony of the penetrating and conception vessels.

Regulation of Emotional and Mental Health

Acne patients should maintain a healthy lifestyle with sufficient sleep and stable emotions. They should also avoid excessive studying, working, or stressful conditions.

CLINICAL EXPERIENCE OF RENOWNED PHYSICIANS

Empirical Formulas

1. Modified *Pí Pá Qīng Fèi Yǐn* (枇杷清肺饮) (Zhu Ren-kang)

【Ingredients】

生地黄	shēng dì huáng	30g	Radix Rehmanniae
牡丹皮	mǔ dān pí	9g	Cortex Moutan
赤芍	chì sháo	9g	Radix Paeoniae Rubra
枇杷叶	pí pá yè	9g	Folium Eriobotryae
桑白皮	sāng bái pí	9g	Cortex Mori
知母	zhī mǔ	9g	Rhizoma Anemarrhenae
黄芩	huáng qín	9g	Radix Scutellariae
生石膏	shēng shí gāo	30g	Gypsum Fibrosum (raw)
生甘草	shēng gān cǎo	6g	Radix et Rhizoma Glycyrrhizae (raw)

【Indications】

Acne associated with lung and stomach accumulated heat.

【Formula Analysis】

Pí pá yè (Folium Eriobotryae), *sāng bái pí* (Cortex Mori), *zhī mǔ* (Rhizoma Anemarrhenae) *huáng qín* (Radix Scutellariae), and *shēng shí gāo* (raw Gypsum Fibrosum) clear and drain lung and stomach fire. *Shēng dì huáng* (Radix Rehmanniae), *mǔ dān pí* (Cortex Moutan), and *chì sháo* (Radix Paeoniae Rubra) clear heat, cool the blood and resolve toxins. *Gān cǎo* (Radix et Rhizoma Glycyrrhizae) clears heat, resolves toxins and harmonizes the actions of other medicinals.

(Guang An Men Hospital of China Academy of Chinese Medical Sciences, *Selected Clinical Cases of Zhu Ren-kang* [朱仁康临床经验集]. Beijing: The People's Medical Publishing House 1986: 194)

2. *Cuò Chuāng Píng* (痤疮平) (Xu Yi-hou)

【Ingredients】

茵陈蒿	yīn chén hāo	15g	Herba Artemisiae Scopariae
白花蛇舌草	bái huā shé shé cǎo	15g	Herba Hedyotis Diffusae
虎杖	hǔ zhàng	15g	Rhizoma Polygoni Cuspidati
蒲公英	pú gōng yīng	15g	Herba Taraxaci
金银花	jīn yín huā	10g	Flos Lonicerae Japonicae
夏枯草	xià kū cǎo	10g	Spica Prunellae
赤芍	chì sháo	10g	Radix Paeoniae Rubra
浙贝母	zhè bèi mǔ	10g	Bulbus Fritillariae Thunbergii
桃仁	táo rén	10g	Semen Persicae
玄参	xuán shēn	10g	Radix Scrophulariae
黄芪	huáng qí	10g	Radix Astragali
紫花地丁	zǐ huā dì dīng	10g	Herba Violae
连翘	lián qiào	10g	Fructus Forsythiae
生石膏	shēng shí gāo	30g	Gypsum Fibrosum (raw)

【Indications】

Acne pustules and nodules. Other signs include a red tongue with a thin yellow coating, and a thready rapid pulse.

【Formula Analysis】

Yīn chén hāo (Herba Artemisiae Scopariae), *bái huā shé shé cǎo* (Herba Hedyotis Diffusae) and *hǔ zhàng* (Rhizoma Polygoni Cuspidati) clear heat, drain dampness and relieve toxins. *Pú gōng yīng* (Herba Taraxaci), *xià kū cǎo* (Spica Prunellae), *xuán shēn* (Radix Scrophulariae), *zhè bèi mǔ* (Bulbus Fritillariae Thunbergii), *zǐ huā dì dīng* (Herba Violae), and *lián qiào* (Fructus Forsythiae) relieve toxins and dissipate nodules. *Chì sháo* (Radix Paeoniae Rubra) and *táo rén* (Semen Persicae) invigorate the blood, transform stasis and dissipate nodules. *Jīn yín huā* (Flos Lonicerae Japonicae) and *shēng shí gāo* (raw Gypsum Fibrosum) clear heat and drain fire to relieve toxins.

(Xu Ai-qin. Experiences of Xu Yi-hou in the Diagnosis and Treatment of Acne (徐宜厚诊疗痤疮经验). *Journal of Traditional Chinese Medicine* (中医杂志),1998, (2):80

3. Píng Cuò Tāng (平痤汤) (Lu De-ming)

【Ingredients】

生地黄	shēng dì huáng	30g	Radix Rehmanniae
玄参	xuán shēn	12g	Radix Scrophulariae
麦门冬	mài mén dōng	9g	Radix Ophiopogonis
天花粉	tiān huā fěn	15g	Radix Trichosanthis
生何首乌	shēng hé shǒu wū	30g	Radix Polygoni multiflori
女贞子	nǚ zhēn zǐ	15g	Fructus Ligustri Lucidi
白花蛇舌草	bái huā shé shé cǎo	30g	Herba Hedyotis Diffusae
丹参	dān shēn	30g	Radix et Rhizoma Salviae Miltiorrhizae
生山楂	shēng shān zhā	30g	Fructus Crataegi (raw)
茶树根	chá shù gēn	30g	Camellia sinensis O. Ktze.
虎杖	hǔ zhàng	15g	Rhizoma Polygoni Cuspidati
苦参	kǔ shēn	12g	Radix Sophorae Flavescentis
黄芩	huáng qín	9g	Radix Scutellariae

【Indications】

Accumulated lung heat leads to toxins ascending to the face. The heat toxin damages yin and thus leads to acne. This formula can clear heat and nourish yin, harmonize the nutritive aspect, and invigorate blood.

(Que Hua-fa. Selected Experiences of Lu De-ming in the Treatment of Acne (陆德铭治痤疮经验撷萃). *Jiangxi Journal of Traditional Chinese Medicine* (江西中医药), 1997, (3): 7)

Selected Case Studies

1. Case Studies of Zhu Ren-kang: Cystic Acne

Mr. Liu, age 21.

【Initial Visit】

January 20th, 1973.

Presenting symptoms: Facial acne with pimples forming cysts for 3 years.

Present history: Over the last three years, facial acne often appeared. Initially this began as acne of the comedo type. The face appears oily with itching and painful pustules and cysts. After the pus was extracted, scars formed. Sometimes they were severe and sometimes mild, however, they did not stop developing nor decrease. After several treatments, the condition still did not improve.

Examination: Localized blackhead acne on the cheeks. Scattered pustules, cysts and atrophic scars developed from the blackheads. On the jaw, there were some scars, knots, and significant seborrhea. There were similar symptoms on the neck, chest and back.

A wiry and slippery pulse, and a red and crimson tongue.

Biomedical diagnosis: Cystic acne.

【Pattern differentiation】

Accumulated heat in the spleen and stomach scorching the lung causes phlegm and stasis, which accumulated for long periods of time resulting in acne.

【Treatment Principle】

Clear heat and cool the blood, disperse phlegm and soften hardness.

【Prescription】

生地黄	shēng dì huáng	30g	Radix Rehmanniae
牡丹皮	mǔ dān pí	9g	Cortex Moutan
赤芍	chì sháo	9g	Radix Paeoniae Rubra
蒲公英	pú gōng yīng	15g	Herba Taraxaci
蚤休	zǎo xiū	60g	Rhizoma Paridis
夏枯草	xià kū cǎo	9g	Spica Prunellae
昆布	kūn bù	9g	Thallus Laminariae
海藻	hǎi zǎo	9g	Sargassum

| 炒三棱 | sān léng | 9g | Rhizoma Sparganii (dry-fried) |
| 炒莪术 | é zhú | 9g | Rhizoma Curcumae (dry-fried) |

The acne improved after 21 doses, with cysts flattened and fewer pustules. At this point the patient began to take pills for the sake of convenience in the long-term course of treatment.

【Prescription】

生地黄	shēng dì huáng	60g	Radix Rehmanniae
丹参	dān shēn	60g	Radix et Rhizoma Salviae Miltiorrhizae
赤芍	chì sháo	60g	Radix Paeoniae Rubra
昆布	kūn bù	30g	Thallus Laminariae
海藻	hǎi zǎo	30g	Sargassum
炒莪术	é zhú	60g	Rhizoma Curcumae (dry-fried)
蒲公英	pú gōng yīng	60g	Herba Taraxaci
蚤休	zǎo xiū	60g	Rhizoma Paridis
夏枯草	xià kū cǎo	60g	Spica Prunellae

Grind the herbs into powder and make into pills using water. Take 9 grams twice a day.

After 2-3 months of treatment, the facial skin had improved markedly and cysts rarely appeared.

(Guang An Men Hospital of China Academy of Chinese Medical Sciences edit. *Clinical Experience Records of Zhu Ren-kang* (朱仁康临床经验集). Beijing: The People's Medical Publishing House, 1986)

2. Case Studies of Lu De-ming: Lung Heat Damaging Yin

Ms. King, age 27.

【Initial Visit】

September 28th, 1994.

Chief complaint: Facial acne for 4 years.

History: In the last 4 years, papules and acnes have consistently occurred on the cheeks and forehead. The acne alternated, sometimes being mild and sometimes being severe. The acne also felt itchy. After squeezing the acne, oily sebum appeared. Despite many attempts at treatment, it had not been cured. Upon examination, there were red papules scattered on the forehead, cheeks, and chin. The tongue was red with a thin coating, and the pulse was slippery.

【Pattern differentiation】

Lung heat damages yin and transforms into heat toxins which ascend to the face.

【Treatment Principle】

Nourish yin and clear heat, harmonize the nutritive aspect and invigorate blood.

【Prescription】

生地黄	shēng dì huáng	30g	Radix Rehmanniae
玄参	xuán shēn	12g	Radix Scrophulariae
麦门冬	mài dōng	9g	Radix Ophiopogonis
天花粉	tiān huā fěn	15g	Radix Trichosanthis
生何首乌	shēng hé shǒu wū	30g	Radix Polygoni multiflori
女贞子	nǚ zhēn zǐ	15g	Fructus Ligustri Lucidi
白花蛇舌草	bái huā shé shé cǎo	30g	Herba Hedyotis Diffusae
丹参	dān shēn	30g	Radix et Rhizoma Salviae Miltiorrhizae
生山楂	shān zhā	30g	Fructus Crataegi (raw)
茶树根	chá shù gēn	30g	Camellia sinensis O. Ktze.
虎杖	hǔ zhàng	15g	Rhizoma Polygoni Cuspidati
苦参	kǔ shēn	12g	Radix Sophorae Flavescentis
黄芩	huáng qín	9g	Radix Scutellariae

There was no significant improvement after taking the prescription for one week. The acne worsened before the menstruation, and then became milder afterward. The patient reported delayed menstruation with scant menses. Tongue coating was thin, and the pulse was slippery.

For these symptoms, *dāng guī* (Radix Angelicae Sinensis), *yì mǔ cǎo* (Herba Leonuri), *yín yáng huò* (Herba Epimedii), and *ròu cōng róng* (Herba

Cistanches) were added to the previous prescription. After three weeks, there was less seborrhea and no itchiness. Continuing for 2 more months, more than half of the acne had disappeared. After another 3 months, the acne was completely healed with no further discomfort.

(Que Hua-fa, Selected Experiences of Lu De-ming in the Treatment of Acne (陆德铭治痤疮经验撷萃), *Jiangxi Journal of Traditional Chinese Medicine* (江西中医药), 1997, (3): 7)

3. Case Studies of Guan Fen: Lung and Stomach Heat

Ms. Lan, age 24.

【Initial Visit】

The patient complained of facial acne for 3 years. There were blackheads and pustules appearing on the face, with oily skin, but no itchiness or pain. Menstruation was reported normal. Upon examination, there were many rashes and blackheads on the face, especially on the forehead, and also some small pustules with local surrounding redness. The tongue was red with a thin coating, and the pulse rapid.

【Pattern differentiation】

Lung and stomach accumulated heat transforming into toxins.

【Treatment Principle】

Clear heat in the lung and stomach, and resolve toxins.

【Prescription】

生石膏	shēng shí gāo	30g	Gypsum Fibrosum (raw)
枇杷叶	pí pá yè	9g	Folium Eriobotryae
桑白皮	sāng bái pí	9g	Cortex Mori
黄芩	huáng qín	9g	Radix Scutellariae
菊花	jú huā	9g	Flos Chrysanthemi
蒲公英	pú gōng yīng	30g	Herba Taraxaci
紫花地丁	zǐ huā dì dīng	30g	Herba Violae
蝉蜕	chán tuì	5g	Periostracum Cicadae

防风	*fáng fēng*	9g	Radix Saposhnikoviae
生甘草	*shēng gān cǎo*	3g	Radix et Rhizoma Glycyrrhizae (raw)

After 20 doses of the prescription, all pustules and rashes disappeared. (Guan Fen. *Practical Dermatology in Chinese Medicine* (实用中医皮肤病学). Lanzhou: Gansu People's Publishing House, 1983:212)

Discussions

1. Zhu Ren-kang on the Two Types of Acne

Zhu Ren-kang theorizes that acne can be divided into two types: lung wind patterns and phlegm stasis patterns. The lung wind pattern is due to the overeating of greasy and rich foods which leads to accumulated heat in the spleen and stomach. The heat ascends to scorch the lung, leaving the lung vulnerable to the invasion of wind evils. This type of acne mainly appears as red rashes, pimples, or small pustules.

A modification of *Pí Pá Qīng Fèi Yǐn* (枇杷清肺饮) is selected to clear lung and stomach heat.

【Prescription】

生地黄	*shēng dì huáng*	30g	Radix Rehmanniae
牡丹皮	*mǔ dān pí*	9g	Cortex Moutan
赤芍	*chì sháo*	9g	Radix Paeoniae Rubra
枇杷叶	*pí pá yè*	9g	Folium Eriobotryae
桑白皮	*sāng bái pí*	9g	Cortex Mori
知母	*zhī mǔ*	9g	Rhizoma Anemarrhenae
黄芩	*huáng qín*	9g	Radix Scutellariae
生石膏	*shēng shí gāo*	30g	Gypsum Fibrosum (raw)
生甘草	*shēng gān cǎo*	6g	Radix et Rhizoma Glycyrrhizae (raw)

The phlegm stasis pattern is caused by phlegm and blood stasis binding together. This type of acne mainly appears with cysts, nodules and scars.

Huà Yū Sàn Jié Wán (化瘀散结丸) is selected to invigorate blood and transform stasis, disperse phlegm, and soften hardness.

【Prescription】

归尾	guī wěi	60g	Radix Angelicae Sinensis (tail)
赤芍	chì sháo	60g	Radix Paeoniae Rubra
桃仁	táo rén	30g	Semen Persicae
红花	hóng huā	30g	Flos Carthami
昆布	kūn bù	30g	Thallus Laminariae
海藻	hǎi zǎo	30g	Sargassum
炒三棱	chǎo sān léng	30g	Rhizoma Sparganii (dry-fried)
炒莪术	chǎo é zhú	30g	Rhizoma Curcumae (dry-fried)
夏枯草	xià kū cǎo	60g	Spica Prunellae
陈皮	chén pí	60g	Pericarpium Citri Reticulatae
制半夏	zhì bàn xià	60g	Rhizoma Pinelliae Praeparatum

Grind the herbs into powder, and mix with water to make pills. 9 grams twice a day.

(Guang An Men Hospital of China Academy of Chinese Medical Sciences. *Clinical Experience Records of Zhu Ren-kang* (朱仁康临床经验集). Beijing: The People's Medical Publishing House 1986.197)

2. Lu De-ming on Hyperactivity of Fire due to Yin Deficiency

Lu De-ming of the Shanghai University of Traditional Chinese Medicine believes that the primary pathogenesis of acne is hyperactivity of fire due to yin deficiency. The secondary causes of acne are accumulated heat in the lung and stomach, and blood stasis in the skin. The main clinical treatment involves nourishing yin and clearing heat. The subsequent treatment principles are to clear heat and invigorate the blood, transform phlegm and soften hardness, and to clear and drain lung-stomach fire.

To nourish yin and clear heat, select *shēng dì huáng* (Radix Rehmanniae), *dān shēn* (Radix et Rhizoma Salviae Miltiorrhizae), *mài dōng* (Radix Ophiopogonis), *tiān huā fěn* (Radix Trichosanthis), *nǚ zhēn zǐ* (Fructus Ligustri Lucidi), *zhī zǐ* (Fructus Gardeniae), and *shēng hé shǒu wū* (Radix

Polygoni multiflori).

To clear heat and resolve toxins, invigorate the blood and dispel stasis, select *bái huā shé shé cǎo* (Herba Hedyotis Diffusae), *hǔ zhàng* (Rhizoma Polygoni Cuspidati), *dān shēn* (Radix et Rhizoma Salviae Miltiorrhizae), *chá shù gēn* (Camellia sinensis O. Ktze) and *shēng shān zhā* (raw Fructus Crataegi).

【Modifications】

➢ For red rashes, add *chì sháo* (Radix Paeoniae Rubra), *mǔ dān pí* (Cortex Moutan), and *lián qiào* (Fructus Forsythiae).

➢ For pustules, add *jīn yín huā* (Flos Lonicerae Japonicae), *bàn zhī lián* (Herba Scutellariae Barbatae), *pú gōng yīng* (Herba Taraxaci), and *yě jú huā* (Flos Chrysanthemi Indici).

➢ For nodules and cysts, add *sān léng* (Rhizoma Sparganii), *é zhú* (Rhizoma Curcumae), *táo rén* (Semen Persicae), *shí jiàn chuān* (Herba Salviae Chinensis), *zào jiǎo cì* (Spina Gleditsiae), *hǎi zǎo* (Sargassum), *xià kū cǎo* (Spica Prunellae), *zhè bèi mǔ* (Bulbus Fritillariae Thunbergii), and *quán guā lóu* (Fructus Trichosanthis).

➢ For itchy rashes, add *kǔ shēn* (Radix Sophorae Flavescentis), *bái xiān pí* (Cortex Dictamni), and *dì fū zǐ* (Fructus Kochiae).

➢ For excessive sebum, add *cè bǎi yè* (Cacumen Platycladi) and *yì yǐ rén* (Semen Coicis).

➢ For hard and dry stools, add *huǒ má rén* (Fructus Cannabis), *yù lǐ rén* (Semen Pruni), *zhǐ shí* (Fructus Aurantii Immaturus), and *dà huáng* (Radix et Rhizoma Rhei).

Clinically, Lu De-ming usually uses *dān shēn* (Radix et Rhizoma Salviae Miltiorrhizae), *bái huā shé shé cǎo* (Herba Hedyotis Diffusae), and *shēng shān zhā* (raw Fructus Crataegi). He believes that the combination of these three herbs regulates the endocrine system, inhibits sebaceous gland secretions, and prevents bacillus (bacterial-type) acne.

(Que Hua-fa. Selected Experiences of Lu De-ming in the Treatment of Acne (陆德铭治痤疮经验撷萃). *Jiangxi Journal of Traditional Chinese Medicine* (江西中医药), 1997, (3):7

3. Xu Yi-hou on "Four Differentiations" and "Ten Treatments" for Acne

Xu Yi-hou of the Wuhan Traditional Chinese Medicine hospital summarizes his clinical experience of acne treatment using the "four differentiations" and "ten treatment methods".

(1) Four Differentiations

1) Differentiating Position

Certain skin conditions are connected to various meridians based on their locations. According to the location and distribution of the channels and collaterals, he finds that skin conditions on the forehead relate to the stomach, around the mouth relates to the spleen, and those appearing on the cheeks relate to the liver. Also, conditions on the chest relate to the conception vessel, where the back relates to the governing vessel.

2) Differentiating Skin Lesions

Blackhead acne is due to dampness predominating over heat, while whitehead acne is due to heat predominating over dampness. Nodules are mostly caused by blood stasis and qi stagnation, while cysts are primarily caused by phlegm-dampness and blood stasis binding together. Pustules are mostly caused by intense heat in the lung and stomach.

3) Differentiating the Physical Constitution

Individuals with weak constitutions and phlegm often belong to patterns of yin deficiency and dryness-heat. Obese individuals often belong to dampness and heat accumulation.

4) Differentiating Subsidiary Symptoms

Xu Yi-hou holds that it is also most important to assess the function of the stomach and large intestine, and in females, the menstruation.

(2) Ten Treatment Methods

Xu Yi-hou summarizes the treatment for acne with ten methods:

1) Clear and drain lung and stomach fire
2) Resolve toxins and dissipate nodules
3) Regulate the penetrating and conception vessels
4) Course the liver and clear heat
5) Invigorate blood and disperse stasis
6) Wet compresses
7) Facial masks
8) Filiform needling
9) Ear acupuncture
10) Pricking method

➤ To clear and drain lung and stomach fire, apply *Bái Hǔ Tāng* (白虎汤) modified with *Pí Pá Qīng Fèi Yǐn* (枇杷清肺饮).

➤ To regulate the penetrating and conception vessels, select *Yì Mǔ Shèng Jīn Dān* (益母胜金丹) with *Èr Xiān Tāng* (二仙汤).

➤ To course the liver and clear heat, select *Dān Zhī Xiāo Yáo Sǎn* (丹栀逍遥散).

➤ To invigorate the blood and disperse stasis, apply modified *Táo Hóng Sì Wù Tāng* (桃红四物汤).

(Xu Ai-qin. Experiences of Xu Yi-hou in the diagnosis and treatment of acne (徐宜厚诊疗痤疮经验), *Journal of Traditional Chinese medicine* (中医杂志), 1998, (2):80)

PERSPECTIVES OF INTEGRATIVE MEDICINE

Challenges and Solutions

The diagnosis of acne is not difficult but treatment is quite challenging due to its frequent recurrence. Acne in women tends to become abundant and severe during the premenstrual period, making the diagnosis and treatment more complex. When acne advances into more severe conditions, it becomes especially hard to cure.

CHALLENGE #1: HOW TO PREVENT RECURRENCE

Acne is a skin disorder associated with dysfunction of the endocrine system. The emotions, psychological state, diet, and intense work or study can all influence the endocrine system. In addition to medical treatment for the prevention of its recurrence, it is important to regulate the mind and emotions and also to improve the diet and lifestyle. Most often, the recurrence of acne in women is related to menstrual irregularities. Therefore, female patients with irregular menstruation are recommended to receive treatment for 3 to 6 months around the menstrual period to reduce or prevent its onset. For married female patients, they could also choose the medication Diane-35, which can regulate menstruation and also cure acne.

CHALLENGE #2: HOW TO TREAT SEVERE ACNE

Severe acne, also known as acne conglobata, mainly manifests with nodules, cysts, pustules, and scarring. If it is not treated properly, it can be most unflattering to the facial appearance and seriously affect the patient's self-image. It is also necessary to examine the patient's endocrine system for any major diseases or problems. Treatment methods include the combining Chinese medical treatment with western biomedicines while also utilizing both internal and external treatments. While treating both root and the branch is essential, treating the root of the problem is most important. Chinese medicine's treatment principles for severe acne include transforming stasis, clearing heat, dispersing phlegm and dissipating nodules.

Typical herbal medicines include *táo rén* (Semen Persicae), *hóng huā* (Flos Carthami), *mǔ dān pí* (Cortex Moutan), *dān shēn* (Radix et

Rhizoma Salviae Miltiorrhizae), *pú gōng yīng* (Herba Taraxaci), *lián qiào* (Fructus Forsythiae), *yù jīn* (Radix Curcumae), *zhè bèi mŭ* (Bulbus Fritillariae Thunbergii), *xuán shēn* (Radix Scrophulariae), *hăi zăo* (Sargassum), and *kūn bù* (Thallus Laminariae). External applications can be used by applying ointments such as *Sì Huáng Gāo* (四黄膏), *Jīn Huáng Gāo* (金黄膏). In western biomedicine, antibiotics such as erythromycin, tetracycline, and clindamycin are often used to treat severe conditions. Combined pharmaceutical approaches using metronidazole, spironolactone and Vitamin B6 have also shown good effects on acne conglobata. Western medications are usually taken for a 1 month period. Then, according to the severity of the acne condition, lower dosages may be applied for 1 to 2 months.

Insight from Empirical Wisdom

1. Treating Acne from the Kidney

In previous decades, many doctors of Chinese medicine believed that the condition of the lung is closely related to the manifestation of acne. They theorized that acne was caused by lung heat and blood heat, and their treatment modality was to clear lung heat, cool blood, and resolve toxins. Through years of clinical experience, it is has been discovered that although acne has some relation with heat in the lung, stomach and blood, the main cause of acne is actually associated with kidney yin deficiency, imbalance of kidney yin-yang, and the hyperactivity of *tian gui* and ministerial fire. In fact, deficient kidney yin leading to hyperactive ministerial fire creates heat in the lung, stomach and blood. Heat then ascends and scorches the face, thus causing acne. Based on this pathomechanism, the proper treatment principle is to nourish the kidney, drain fire, clear the lung, and resolve toxins.

The formula that best meets this treatment principle is *Xiāo Cuò Tāng*

(消痤汤). This formula is a modified version of the traditional formulas *Zhī Bǎi Dì Huáng Wán* (知柏地黄丸) and *Èr Zhì Wán* (二至丸).

Ingredients in *Xiāo Cuò Tāng* (消痤汤) include: *zhī mǔ* (Rhizoma Anemarrhenae) 12g, *huáng bǎi* (Cortex Phellodendri Chinensis) 12g, *nǚ zhēn zǐ* (Fructus Ligustri Lucidi) 20g, *hàn lián cǎo* (Herba Ecliptae) 20g, *shēng dì huáng* (Radix Rehmanniae) 15g, *yú xīng cǎo* (Herba Houttuyniae) 20g, *pú gōng yīng* (Herba Taraxaci) 20g, *lián qiào* (Fructus Forsythiae) 15g, *dān shēn* (Radix et Rhizoma Salviae Miltiorrhizae) 25g, and *gān cǎo* (Radix et Rhizoma Glycyrrhizae) 5g.

More recently, a new theory to treat acne from the liver has been developed. This is rooted in the theory that acne is associated with the kidney. The liver and kidney are of the same source, the kidney dominates water, and the liver belongs to wood. If kidney yin is deficient, then water cannot nourish wood. Thus, liver yin will become deficient as well, and it will fail to maintain the normal flow of qi. Consequently, liver fire may rise to create acne or aggravate current conditions. Based on this theory, it is most essential to adopt the treatment principles of regulating the liver and kidney, enriching the kidney, and purging the liver.

2. DĀN SHĒN (RADIX ET RHIZOMA SALVIAE MILTIORRHIZAE) AND ACNE TREATMENT

Dān shēn (Radix et Rhizoma Salviae Miltiorrhizae) has the properties of bitterness and slight coldness. These properties can dispel blood stasis, relieve pain, cool and invigorate the blood, clear the heart, and eliminate vexation. Using *dān shēn* (Radix et Rhizoma Salviae Miltiorrhizae) (30-50g each time) in large dosages when combined with other herbs can effectively treat recurrent acne with cysts, nodules, and scarring. Because *dān shēn* (Radix et Rhizoma Salviae Miltiorrhizae) invigorates the blood, it should be removed from some formulas, or used in small dosages for women during menstruation. However, it is appropriate to use large doses of *dān shēn* (Radix et Rhizoma Salviae Miltiorrhizae) for acne patients with delayed menstruation when caused by qi stagnation and blood stasis combined with heat. When patients have painful menstruation due to stasis and heat binding together or disharmony of the penetrating and conception vessels, it is then appropriate to apply *dān shēn* (Radix et Rhizoma Salviae Miltiorrhizae) with *chái hú* (Radix Bupleuri), *yù jīn* (Radix Curcumae), *yì mǔ cǎo* (Herba Leonuri), and *xiāng fù* (Rhizoma Cyperi).

3. Perspectives of Integrative Medicine

Both Chinese medicine and biomedicine have their own advantages in the treatment of acne. Chinese medicine emphasizes healing from a more holistic point of view. It also displays less side effects, and the combining of internal and external treatments are typically applied. Clinical practice indicates that treating severe acne by integrating Chinese medicine with western medicine is the best approach. The author treats mild cases of acne with Chinese medicine alone, however. For severe cases such as acne conglobata and acne scrofulosorum, he combines Chinese medicinals with western drugs including antibiotics, retinol, and anti-androgen medications for short-term treatment. When the acne condition improves, he withdraws the western medications and uses only Chinese medicine to consolidate the effect. Chinese medicine can also reduce side effects of the long-term use of antibiotics and retinol.

Summary

Acne is skin condition quite commonly seen in clinic. As it primarily affects the face, many individuals feel self-conscious and actively seek out treatments to improve their appearance. The treatment of acne with Chinese medicine has progressed significantly in the last ten years. The standard etiologies of acne have now expanded beyond the traditional categories of wind heat, lung heat, and blood heat to also include patterns of damp-heat, blood stasis, phlegm bind, insufficient kidney yin, and hyperactivity of the ministerial fire. These new perspectives have given new direction and meaning to the clinical treatment of acne. Various new treatments have been developed such as treating the kidney, blood, blood stasis, or phlegm to cure acne, which have achieved good clinical results. Acne is an interior disease that appears on the exterior, and thus it is important to treat both internally and externally, and the root and branch simultaneously. In clinical practice, a combined therapy using both internal treatments and external applications has shown greater superiority than the individual therapies applied separately.

Presently, there is a great amount of medical literature on Chinese medicine's treatment of acne. However, there is only a small minority of high quality research due to poor adherence to proper clinical research design. Although many medical journals report clinical cases, there are very few research studies with randomized control groups. Results from these reports do not have unified standards and therefore show little reliability in demonstrating a curative effect. Some acne treatments do not have a standard method of comparison to measure true efficacy. Lab studies on the Chinese medicine treatment of acne are rarely conducted and thus cannot scientifically explain how Chinese medicine can cure acne. Since there is currently no effective western medication to treat acne, the prospect of using Chinese medicine to cure acne is bright.

Research on Chinese medicine for treating acne can further develop by advancing Chinese medical theory, increasing the use of patent medicines, and adopting modern medical science. First, there should be a strong focus on medical research on the use of Chinese medicine in order to develop new theories and treatments. For example, treating the kidney or liver to cure acne may be a worthwhile research topic. Secondly, there should be serious consideration in researching Chinese patent medicine for acne. Acne is a very common dermatological disease, and in order to cure it, patients need to take medicine frequently. Chinese patent medicine may be a great option because of its excellent results, lack of side effects, and its convenience in today's modern society. Thirdly, it is also imperative to use modern medical science and proper research methodologies to improve and substantiate the effects of Chinese medicine in its treatment of acne. Other medical disciplines such as endocrinology, immunology, molecular biology, microbiology, and pathology may eventually corroborate and contribute its findings to Chinese medicine's method of treating acne. This interdisciplinary approach would certainly raise Chinese medicine to a higher level of academic and scientific standard.

SELECTED QUOTES FROM CLASSICAL TEXTS

Discussion of the Origins of the Symptoms of Disease—Category of Acne on the Face (诸病源候论·面疱候 , *Zhū Bìng Yuán Hòu Lùn: Miàn Pào Hòu*):
面疱者，谓面上有风热气生疮，头如米大，白色者是。
"Facial acne can appear with sores that are white and the size of a rice grain. This is caused by wind heat affecting the face."

Orthodox Lineage of External Medicine 81—Lung Wind, Acne and Rosacea (外科正宗· 肺风粉刺酒渣鼻第八十一 , *Wài Kē Zhèng Zōng: Fèi Fēng Fěn Cì Jiǔ Zhā Bí Dì Bā Shí Yī*):
肺风、粉刺、酒渣鼻三名同种。粉刺属肺，渣鼻属脾，总皆血热郁滞不散。
"Lung wind, acne, and rosacea are three different names for the same disease. Acne belongs to the lung, and rosacea belongs to the spleen. Both are caused by the stagnation of heat in blood. "

Enlightenment on the Mystery of External Medicine (外科启玄 , *Wài Kē Qǐ Xuán*):

妇女面生窠瘘作痒，名曰粉花疮。乃肺受风热或绞面感风，致生粉刺，盖受湿热也。

"Acne on a woman's face which is itchy is referred to as a flower sore. It is caused by wind heat invading the lung or wind invading the face during facial hair removal. These are both related to damp-heat."

Golden Mirror of the Medical Tradition—Essential Rhymes of the Heart-Approach in External Medicine (医宗金鉴·外科心法要诀, *Yī Zōng Jīn Jiàn: Wài Kē Xīn Fǎ Yào Jué*):

肺风粉刺，此病由肺经血热而成。

"Lung wind acne is caused by blood heat in the lung channel."

MODERN RESEARCH

Clinical Research

1. Pattern Differentiation and Corresponding Treatment

Chinese medicine differentiates acne into different patterns according to its etiology, pathogenesis, symptoms and signs. Common patterns reported in the literature include blood heat in the lung and stomach, damp-heat in the spleen and stomach, yin deficiency generating interior heat, disharmony of the penetrating and conception vessels, stasis-phlegm bind, spleen deficiency, and phlegm-dampness.

2. Treatment

There are several clinical approaches which include internal treatments, external treatments, and the integration of both internal and external treatments. Of these three, the combined treatment method is the most common and most effective approach.

(1) Internal Treatment

For internal treatment, doctors usually select a formula according to the presenting pattern. Commonly used prescriptions include *Pí Pá Qīng Fèi Yǐn* (枇杷清肺饮), *Xiè Bái Sǎn* (泻白散), *Lóng Dǎn Xiè Gān Tāng* (龙胆泻肝汤), *Yīn Chén Hāo Tāng* (茵陈蒿汤), *Wǔ Wèi Qīng Dú Yǐn* (五味清毒饮), *Huáng Lián Jiě Dú Tāng* (黄连解毒汤), *Táo Hóng Sì Wù Tāng* (桃红四物汤), *Dān Zhī Xiāo Yáo Sǎn* (丹栀逍遥散), *Èr Zhì Wán* (二至丸), *Zhī Bǎi Bā Wèi Wán* (知柏八味丸).

Empirical formulas composed by individual doctors include *Xiāo Cuò Tāng* (消痤汤), *Xiāo Cuò Yǐn* (消痤饮), *Cuò Chuāng Yǐn* (痤疮饮), *Xiāo Chuāng Měi Róng Tāng* (消疮美容汤), *Cuò Chuāng Píng* (痤疮平), and *Qīng Fèi Xiāo Dú Yǐn* (清肺消毒饮). All of these are widely used in clinic, some of which have been adapted to modern forms of medication such as liquid, powders, tablets, and capsules.

1) Pattern Differentiation and Choice of Formula

Li Zheng divided acne into four types:

A. Accumulated Heat in the Lung and Stomach

Main symptoms: red papules, blushing, oily face, pain or itchiness.

Treat with modifications of *Pí Pá Qīng Fèi Yǐn* (枇杷清肺饮): *pí pá yè* (Folium Eriobotryae), *sāng bái pí* (Cortex Mori), *huáng qín* (Radix Scutellariae), *zhī zǐ* (Fructus Gardeniae), *mǔ dān pí* (Cortex Moutan), *chē qián cǎo* (Herba Plantaginis), *bái máo gēn* (Rhizoma Imperatae), and *shēng shí gāo* (raw Gypsum Fibrosum) to clear damp-heat in the lung and stomach and cool the blood to eliminate papules.

B. Excess Heat Transforming into Toxins

Main symptoms: red lesions with pus, hot and burning pain.

Treat with modifications of *Wǔ Wèi Xiāo Dú Yǐn* (五味消毒饮): *jīn yín huā* (Flos Lonicerae Japonicae), *lián qiào* (Fructus Forsythiae), *pú gōng yīng* (Herba Taraxaci), *zǐ huā dì dīng* (Herba Violae), *yě jú huā* (Flos

Chrysanthemi Indici), *pí pá yè* (Folium Eriobotryae), *zhī zǐ* (Fructus Gardeniae), *xuán shēn* (Radix Scrophulariae), and *huáng qín* (Radix Scutellariae) to clear heat, relieve toxins, unblock *fu* organs, and eliminate stagnation.

C. Disharmony of the Penetrating and Conception Vessels

Main symptoms: dark red lesions which are worse before menstruation and generally alleviated after menstruation. Irregular menstruation or lower abdominal pain before menstruation.

Treated with modifications of *Sì Wù Tāng* (四物汤) plus *Pí Pá Qīng Fèi Yǐn* (枇杷清肺饮): *shēng dì huáng* (Radix Rehmanniae), *chì sháo* (Radix Paeoniae Rubra), *bái sháo* (Radix Paeoniae Alba), *dāng guī* (Radix Angelicae Sinensis), *chuān xiōng* (Rhizoma Chuanxiong), *nǚ zhēn zǐ* (Fructus Ligustri Lucidi), *hàn lián cǎo* (Herba Ecliptae), *dì gǔ pí* (Cortex Lycii), and *pí pá yè* (Folium Eriobotryae) to harmonize the penetrating and conception vessels and to clear heat in the lung.

D. Blood Stasis and Phlegm Congestion

Main symptoms: dark red lesions, cysts or nodules, scarring, and local pain or itching. It should be treated with modifications of *Táo Hóng Sì Wù Tāng* (桃红四物汤) plus *Èr Chén Tāng* (二陈汤): *dāng guī* (Radix Angelicae Sinensis), *chì sháo* (Radix Paeoniae Rubra), *táo rén* (Semen Persicae), *hóng huā* (Flos Carthami), *shēng dì huáng* (Radix Rehmanniae), *chuān xiōng* (Rhizoma Chuanxiong), *xiāng fù* (Rhizoma Cyperi), *zhì bàn xià* (Rhizoma Pinelliae Praeparatum), *jú pí* (Pericarpium Citri Reticulatae), *fú líng* (Poria), *bái jiāng cán* (Bombyx Batryticatus), *xià kū cǎo* (Spica Prunellae), and *lián qiào* (Fructus Forsythiae) to invigorate the blood and regulate qi, transform phlegm and dissipate nodules.

The first and second decoctions may be taken orally, and a third decoction may be used as a cold compress. In total, 136 cases were treated with a 95.59% rate of efficacy.[1]

Zhang Hong-ya divided acne into three types:

A. Wind Heat in the Lung Channel

Treat with *Pí Pá Qīng Fèi Yǐn* (枇杷清肺饮) plus *Yīn Chén Hāo Tāng* (茵陈蒿汤): *huáng qín* (Radix Scutellariae), *zhī zǐ* (Fructus Gardeniae), *chuān xiōng* (Rhizoma Chuanxiong), *shēng gān cǎo* (raw Radix et Rhizoma Glycyrrhizae), *yīn chén hāo* (Herba Artemisiae Scopariae), *sāng bái pí* (Cortex Mori), *pí pá yè* (Folium Eriobotryae), and *shēng dà huáng* (raw Radix et Rhizoma Rhei) to diffuse the lung, eliminate wind and clear heat.

B. Damp Heat in the Lung and Stomach

Treat with modifications of *Yīn Chén Hāo Tāng* (茵陈蒿汤): *yīn chén hāo* (Herba Artemisiae Scopariae), *huáng qín* (Radix Scutellariae), *zhī zǐ* (Fructus Gardeniae), *cāng zhú* (Rhizoma Atractylodis), *bái zhú* (Rhizoma Atractylodis Macrocephalae), *dà qīng yè* (Folium Isatidis), *fú líng* (Poria), *zé xiè* (Rhizoma Alismatis), and *shēng dà huáng* (raw Radix et Rhizoma Rhei) to clear heat, drain dampness, and unblock the *fu* organs.

C. Qi Stagnation and Blood Stasis

Treat with *Táo Hóng Sì Wù Tāng* (桃红四物汤): *quán dāng guī* (Radix Angelicae Sinensis), *shēng dì huáng* (Radix Rehmanniae), *chì sháo* (Radix Paeoniae Rubra), *bái sháo* (Radix Paeoniae Alba), *chuān xiōng* (Rhizoma Chuanxiong), *táo rén* (Semen Persicae), *hóng huā* (Flos Carthami), *dān shēn* (Radix et Rhizoma Salviae Miltiorrhizae), *yīn chén hāo* (Herba Artemisiae Scopariae), and *xià kū cǎo* (Spica Prunellae) to regulate qi, invigorate the blood, and eliminate stasis. In total, 69 cases were treated with a 94.02% rate of efficacy.[2]

Feng Jian-hua believes that pattern differentiation involves the lung, heart, liver, spleen, stomach and kidney. Based on clinical observation and diagnosis, acne is divided into five types: lung heat, heart and liver fire, damp heat in stomach and intestine, heat toxin with stasis, and phlegm and stasis bind.

A. Lung Heat

Treat with modifications of *Pí Pá Qīng Fèi Yǐn* (枇杷清肺饮) plus *Qīng Yíng Tāng* (清营汤): *pí pá yè* (Folium Eriobotryae) 10g, *sāng bái pí* (Cortex Mori) 15-30g, *huáng qín* (Radix Scutellariae) 12g, *mǔ dān pí* (Cortex Moutan) 10g, *zhī zǐ* (Fructus Gardeniae) 9g, *yě jú huā* (Flos Chrysanthemi Indici) 9g, *shēng dì huáng* (Radix Rehmanniae) 15g, *lián qiào* (Fructus Forsythiae) 15g, *xuán shēn* (Radix Scrophulariae) 15g, *shuǐ niú jiǎo* (Cornu Bubali) 60g, *dān shēn* (Radix et Rhizoma Salviae Miltiorrhizae) 15g, *dàn zhú yè* (Herba Lophatheri) 9g, and *shēng gān cǎo* (raw Radix et Rhizoma Glycyrrhizae) 9g to purge the lung and clear heat, cool the blood, and resolve toxins.

B. Heart and Liver Fire

Treat with modifications of *Dāng Guī Lú Huì Wán* (当归芦荟丸), *Xiè Xīn Tāng* (泻心汤) and *Jiā Wèi Xiāo Yáo Sǎn* (加味逍遥散): *dāng guī* (Radix Angelicae Sinensis) 12g, *lú huì* (Aloe) 2-3g (take directly after mixing with hot water), *huáng lián* (Rhizoma Coptidis) 9g, *huáng qín* (Radix Scutellariae) 10g, *lóng dǎn cǎo* (Radix Gentianae) 9g, *chái hú* (Radix Bupleuri) 9g, *mǔ dān pí* (Cortex Moutan) 10g, *zhī zǐ* (Fructus Gardeniae) 9g, *lián qiào* (Fructus Forsythiae) 15g, *shēng dì huáng* (Radix Rehmanniae) 15g, *xuán shēn* (Radix Scrophulariae) 15g, *chì sháo* (Radix Paeoniae Rubra) 12g, *xiāng fù* (Rhizoma Cyperi) 9g, and *shēng gān cǎo* (raw Radix et Rhizoma Glycyrrhizae) 9g to clear liver and drain fire, cool the blood, and resolve toxins.

With symptoms of liver constraint syndrome such as irritability and sleeplessness, fullness in the chest and hypochondriac region, breast tenderness and distention before menstruation, and irregular menstruation, it is appropriate to course the liver, resolve constraint, invigorate the blood, and regulate menstruation with modifications of *Jiā Wèi Xiāo Yáo Sǎn* (加味逍遥散) plus *Táo Hóng Sì Wù Tāng* (桃红四物汤): *chái hú* (Radix Bupleuri) 9g, *bái sháo* (Radix Paeoniae Alba) 12g, *mǔ dān pí* (Cortex Moutan) 12g, *zhī zǐ* (Fructus Gardeniae) 10g, *dāng guī* (Radix Angelicae Sinensis) 15g, *xiāng fù* (Rhizoma Cyperi) 9g, *chuān xiōng* (Rhizoma Chuanxiong) 9g, *zhǐ qiào* (Fructus Aurantii) 9g, *táo rén* (Semen Persicae) 9g, *hóng huā* (Flos Carthami) 9g, and *pú gōng yīng* (Herba Taraxaci) 15g.

C. Damp-heat in the Intestine and Stomach

Treat by clearing heat, resolving toxins, unblocking the *fu* organs, and draining dampness with modifications of *Qīng Wèi Sǎn* (清胃散): *huáng lián* (Rhizoma Coptidis) 9g, *mǔ dān pí* (Cortex Moutan) 10g, *zhī zǐ* (Fructus Gardeniae) 9g, *jīn yín huā* (Flos Lonicerae Japonicae) 20g, *lián qiào* (Fructus Forsythiae) 15g, *lóng dǎn cǎo* (Radix Gentianae) 9g, *shēng má* (Rhizoma Cimicifugae) 9g, *xuán shēn* (Radix Scrophulariae) 15g, *pèi lán* (Herba Eupatorii) 9g, *hé yè* (Folium Nelumbinis) 9g, *zé xiè* (Rhizoma Alismatis) 12g, *shēng dà huáng* (raw Radix et Rhizoma Rhei) 6g, and *shēng gān cǎo* (raw Radix et Rhizoma Glycyrrhizae) 9g.

D. Heat Toxins with Stasis

Treat with methods that clear heat, resolve toxins, invigorate the blood and transform stasis with modifications of *Sān Huáng Shí Gāo Tāng* (三黄石膏汤) plus *Wǔ Wèi Xiāo Dú Yǐn* (五味消毒饮): *huáng qín* (Radix Scutellariae) 12g, *huáng lián* (Rhizoma Coptidis) 9g, *huáng bǎi* (Cortex Phellodendri Chinensis) 9g, *zhī zǐ* (Fructus Gardeniae) 10g, *shēng shí gāo* (raw Gypsum Fibrosum) 30g, *jīn yín huā* (Flos Lonicerae Japonicae) 30g, *yě jú huā* (Flos Chrysanthemi Indici) 9g, *pú gōng yīng* (Herba Taraxaci) 15g, *zǐ huā dì dīng* (Herba Violae) 12g, *dāng guī* (Radix Angelicae Sinensis) 15g, *táo rén* (Semen Persicae) 9g, *hóng huā* (Flos Carthami) 9g, *zé lán* (Herba Lycopi) 9g, *shēng dà huáng* (raw Radix et Rhizoma Rhei) 6g, and *shēng gān cǎo* (raw Radix et Rhizoma Glycyrrhizae) 9g.

E. Phlegm and Stasis Bind

Treat with methods that transform phlegm, dissipate nodules, invigorate blood, and eliminate stasis with modifications of *Táo*

Hóng Sì Wù Tāng (桃红四物汤) plus *Fú Líng Wán* (茯苓丸): *dāng guī* (Radix Angelicae Sinensis) 15g, *xiāng fù* (Rhizoma Cyperi) 9g, *chuān xiōng* (Rhizoma Chuanxiong) 9g, *táo rén* (Semen Persicae) 9g, *hóng huā* (Flos Carthami) 9g, *sān léng* (Rhizoma Sparganii) 12g, *é zhú* (Rhizoma Curcumae) 12g, *mǔ dān pí* (Cortex Moutan) 10g, *fú líng* (Poria) 15g, *zhì bàn xià* (Rhizoma Pinelliae Praeparatum) 9g, *dǎn nán xīng* (Arisaema cum Bile) 9g, *kūn bù* (Thallus Laminariae) 30g, *hé yè* (Folium Nelumbinis) 9g, *zhè bèi mǔ* (Bulbus Fritillariae Thunbergii) 12g, and *mǔ lì* (Concha Ostreae) 30g.[3]

2) Specific Formulas

Xiong Ya-li believes that the main pathogenesis of acne is accumulated heat in the lung and stomach. Dr. Xiong used *Yù Nǚ Jiān* (玉女煎), derived from *Collected Treatises of [Zhang] Jing-yue* (景岳全书, *Jǐng Yuè Quán Shū*). Modifications are applied to clear and drain the lung and stomach, and downbear fire toxins: *shēng dì huáng* (Radix Rehmanniae), *shēng shí gāo* (raw Gypsum Fibrosum), *yě jú huā* (Flos Chrysanthemi Indici), *zhī mǔ* (Rhizoma Anemarrhenae), *chì sháo* (Radix Paeoniae Rubra), *niú xī* (Radix Achyranthis Bidentatae), *huáng qín* (Radix Scutellariae), and *gān cǎo* (Radix et Rhizoma Glycyrrhizae).

In total, 120 cases were treated with a 90.84% rate of efficacy.[4]

Han Yong-sheng believes that the cause of acne is mainly blood heat and wind heat in the lung channel. Therefore, he chose modifications of *Pí Pá Qīng Fèi Yǐn* (枇杷清肺饮): *pí pá yè* (Folium Eriobotryae), *huáng lián* (Rhizoma Coptidis), *huáng qín* (Radix Scutellariae), *wū méi* (Fructus Mume), *sāng bái pí* (Cortex Mori), *gān cǎo* (Radix et Rhizoma Glycyrrhizae), *yì yǐ rén* (Semen Coicis), *bǎi bù* (Radix Stemonae), *bái huā shé shé cǎo* (Herba Hedyotis Diffusae), *táo rén* (Semen Persicae), and *hóng huā* (Flos Carthami).

This formula treated 120 cases of acne. All cases, except one, had positive outcomes.[5]

Xu Xin used modifications of *Pǔ Jì Xiāo Dú Yǐn* (普济消毒饮) to treat 50 subjects with acne. Of these subjects, 30 cases were cured, 11 cases improved, and 1 case had no effect. The rate of effectiveness was 98.0%.

The herbs in the basic formula were: *huáng qín* (Radix Scutellariae) 10g, *huáng lián* (Rhizoma Coptidis) 6g, *chén pí* (Pericarpium Citri Reticulatae) 10g, *xuán shēn* (Radix Scrophulariae) 20g, *jié gěng* (Radix Platycodonis) 10g, *bǎn lán gēn* (Radix Isatidis) 30g, *shēng má* (Rhizoma Cimicifugae) 10g, *mǎ bó* (Lasiosphaera seu Calvatia) 10g, *lián qiào* (Fructus Forsythiae) 12g, *niú bàng zǐ* (Fructus Arctii) 10g, *bò hé* (Herba Menthae) 10g (decocted later), *bái jiāng cán* (Bombyx Batryticatus) 10g, *shēng yì yǐ rén* (raw Semen Coicis) 30g, and *gān cǎo* (Radix et Rhizoma Glycyrrhizae) 10g.

Patients were instructed to decoct one bag of herbs to be divided and taken twice a day. One course of treatment equaled 10 days. Patients were allowed a maximum of five courses of treatment.[6]

Yang Wen-xin applied an empirical formula named *Yùn Pí Sàn Jié Tāng* (运脾散结汤) to treat 712 cases of recurring acne. Results showed 472 cases cured (66.3%), 194 cases improved, and 46 cases with no effective outcome. The rate of effectiveness for both the cured and improved cases was 93%.

The herbs in the formula were: *dǎng shēn* (Radix Codonopsis) 15g, *biǎn dòu* (Semen Dolichoris Lablab) 15g, *shān zhā* (Fructus Crataegi) 15g, *yīn chén* (Herba Artemisiae Scopariae) 12g, *bái zhú* (Rhizoma Atractylodis Macrocephalae) 12g, *pí pá yè* (Folium Eriobotryae) 15g, *fáng fēng* (Radix Saposhnikoviae) 12g, and *zhè bèi mǔ* (Bulbus Fritillariae Thunbergii) 12g.

➤ For pustules, add *pú gōng yīng* (Herba Taraxaci) and *zǐ huā dì dīng* (Herba Violae).

➤ For the hardening of tissue, add *sān léng* (Rhizoma Sparganii) and *é zhú* (Rhizoma Curcumae).

➤ For small itchy lesions, add *bǎi bù* (Radix Stemonae).

The patient should take one bag of the above formula per day. Decoct one bag three times in water until 300 ml of the decoction is left. To be taken three times a day.

Twenty days constitute one course of treatment. One treatment cycle consists of two full courses of treatment (a total of 40 days).[7]

Liang Shang-cai used modifications of *Fěn Cì Jiān* (粉刺煎) to treat acne: *pí pá yè* (Folium Eriobotryae), *huáng qín* (Radix Scutellariae), *sāng bái pí* (Cortex Mori), *chì sháo* (Radix Paeoniae Rubra), *bái huā shé shé cǎo* (Herba Hedyotis Diffusae), *lián qiào* (Fructus Forsythiae), *mǔ dān pí* (Cortex Moutan), *shēng shān zhā* (raw Fructus Crataegi), *shēng dì huáng* (Radix Rehmanniae), *zhī zǐ* (Fructus Gardeniae), *tiān huā fěn* (Radix Trichosanthis), *yě jú huā* (Flos Chrysanthemi Indici), *yì yǐ rén* (Semen Coicis), etc. One bag of this formula should be taken once per day for ten days as one course of treatment.

Of the 240 cases, the recovery rate was 60%, and the total effective rate was 97.5%.[8]

Yang En-pin wrote a formula named *Cuò Chuāng Qīng Xiāo Yǐn* (痤疮清消饮): *pí pá yè* (Folium Eriobotryae), *shēng sāng bái pí* (raw Cortex Mori), *yù jīn* (Radix Curcumae), *chóng lóu* (Rhizoma Paridis), *lián qiào* (Fructus Forsythiae), *rěn dōng téng* (Caulis Lonicerae Japonicae), *shēng dì huáng* (Radix Rehmanniae), *mǔ dān pí* (Cortex Moutan), *chǎo huáng qín* (dry-fried Radix Scutellariae), and *huáng lián* (Rhizoma Coptidis). This formula was used to treat 102 cases of acne. The formula should be taken twice a day, once each morning and evening. One bag of herbs may be used for 2 days.

Four weeks constituted one course of treatment. The total rate of effectiveness was 95%.[9]

(2) External Treatment

In addition to acupuncture and other topical applications, there are numerous ways of treating externally. Besides tinctures, liquids, and powders, there are also new forms of treatment using creams, serums, and facial masks.

1) Chinese Medicinal Facial Mask

The Chinese medicinal facial mask is a new external treatment which combines concentrated Chinese medicinals and massage. It provides a slightly warming therapy, cleans the skin in the deep layers, and promotes transdermal absorption of Chinese medicine into the facial skin. This method has shown good effect on facial skin conditions such as acne.

Yang Ying-cheng used a Chinese medicinal facial mask to treat 130 cases of acne. After two courses of therapy, the recovery rate was 91.5% and the total effective rate was 99.2%.[10]

The facial mask ingredients are: *liú huáng* (Sulfur) 5g, *dà huáng* (Radix et Rhizoma Rhei) 5g, *huáng bǎi* (Cortex Phellodendri Chinensis) 5g, *bò hé* (Herba Menthae) 6g, *jú huā* (Flos Chrysanthemi) 6g, *mǔ lì* (Concha Ostreae) 6g, *kū fán* (Alumen) 10g, *huáng lián* (Rhizoma Coptidis) 4g, and *bīng piàn* (Borneolum Syntheticum) 1g.

Grind all the medicinals into a very fine powder. Take 2g of the powder and mix with 5g cream to make a paste-like substance. After cleaning and massaging the face, apply the paste. Then apply as a gypsum mask, using *shí gāo* (Gypsum Fibrosum), and remove the mask 25 minutes later. The mask should be applied once every 6 days for 1 month, which constitutes one course of treatment.

After 2 courses of treatment, the recovery rate was 91.5% and the total rate of effectiveness was 99.2%.[10]

Yan Lu-juan developed a facial mask for the treatment of 36 acne cases. After 10 treatments, the recovery rate was 57.5% and the total rate of effectiveness was 97.5%. The facial mask ingredients include: *dān shēn*

(Radix et Rhizoma Salviae Miltiorrhizae) 40g, *dà huáng* (Radix et Rhizoma Rhei) 20g, *bái huā shé shé cǎo* (Herba Hedyotis Diffusae) 20g, and *yì yǐ rén* (Semen Coicis) 20g.[11]

Shi Ping developed a Chinese medicinal facial mask for the treatment of 55 cases of acne. Twenty-nine subjects were cured, 17 cases improved, 6 cases showed a slight effect, and 3 cases had no effect. The total rate of effectiveness was 83%.

The facial mask ingredients include: *huáng lián* (Rhizoma Coptidis) 10g, *huáng qín* (Radix Scutellariae) 10g, *dān shēn* (Radix et Rhizoma Salviae Miltiorrhizae) 10g, *bái jí* (Bletilla striata) 10g, *lú huì* (Aloe) 10g, *jīn yín huā* (Flos Lonicerae Japonicae) *10g, fú líng* (Poria) 10g, *dān pí* (Cortex Moutan) 10g, *dāng guī* (Radix Angelicae Sinensis) 10g, *jiāng huáng* (Rhizoma Curcumae Longae) 10g, *bái huā shé shé cǎo* (Herba Hedyotis Diffusae) 15g, and *xìng rén* (Semen Armeniacae Amarum).

First, grind the herbs into a fine powder. Second, mix 100g of the powder with 250g of sesame oil to create a massage cream. Third, mix 200g of gypsum powder (using *shēng shí gāo* (raw Gypsum Fibrosum)) with 50g of the herbal medicine powder to create a facial mask powder.

First, clean the skin, and apply to the face a thin uniform layer of Chinese medicinal massage cream, and gently massage the face for 15-20 minutes along the channels. Then spray the face with a negative ion spray. Second, mix the facial mask powder with warm water to make a paste. Apply the paste evenly (avoiding the eyes, nose and mouth). Remove 30 minutes later, and clean the face. Repeat this regimen once every two days for one week.[12]

2) Fuming and Washing

Ren Zhi-min created an empirical decoction for the treatment of acne. The ingredients include *kǔ shēn* (Radix Sophorae Flavescentis) 30g, *mǔ dān pí* (Cortex Moutan) 30g, *lóng dǎn cǎo* (Radix Gentianae) 30g, *pú gōng yīng* (Herba Taraxaci) 30g, *wū yā téng gēn* 30g, *dì fū zǐ* (Fructus Kochiae) 20g, and *dà qīng yè* (Folium Isatidis) 20g. Decoct the herbs with water over low heat for 20-30 minutes. The decoction is used for facial steaming and washing. It should be applied twice a day for 10 days as one course of treatment, with 5 days between each course.

The rate of effectiveness was 91.18%.[13]

Wang Xiao-hong created an empirical herbal formula called *Cuò Yù Sǎn* (痤愈散) which includes: *dà huáng* (Radix et Rhizoma Rhei) 20g, *kǔ shēn* (Radix Sophorae Flavescentis) 20g, *jīng jiè* (Herba Schizonepetae) 20g, *máng xiāo* (Natrii Sulfas) 20g, *zǐ cǎo* (Radix Arnebiae) 20g, *cè bǎi yè* (Cacumen Platycladi) 20g, and *dāng guī wěi* (Radix Angelicae Sinensis) 20g. Grind into powder and place into a small gauze pouch. Then place the pouch into 500ml of water and boil. Steam the face for 30 minutes. Be sure to keep sufficient distance from the steam to avoid burning. Apply once daily.

The rate of effectiveness was 99.8%.[14]

Yu Gui-tian created an empirical facial wash using *tù sī zǐ* (Semen Cuscutae). Decoct 30g in 500ml of water, until 300ml remains. The decoction was applied to the affected areas 1-2 times a day for 7 days, which constituted a single course of treatment.

With 1-2 courses of treatment, 50 cases of acne were effectively treated at a 94% success rate.[15]

3) Dressing

Zhang Lei used *Jīn Huáng Sǎn* (金黄散) to treat 100 cases of facial acne. Its cure rate was 67% and total effective rate was 88%.

Grind the following herbs into a fine powder: *tiān huā fěn* (Radix Trichosanthis) 250g, *dà huáng* (Radix et Rhizoma Rhei) 250g, *bái zhǐ* (Radix Angelicae Dahuricae) 250g, *huáng bǎi* (Cortex Phellodendri Chinensis) 250g, *jiāng huáng* (Rhizoma Curcumae Longae) 250g, *jú pí* (Pericarpium

Citri Reticulatae) 100g, *hòu pò* (Cortex Magnoliae Officinalis) 100g, *cāng zhú* (Rhizoma Atractylodis) 100g, *dǎn nán xīng* (Arisaema cum Bile) 100g, and *gān cǎo* (Radix et Rhizoma Glycyrrhizae) 100g. Filter the powder through an 80 mesh screen sieve. Then add *xióng huáng* (Realgar) 100g, *bīng piàn* (Borneolum Syntheticum), and *bò hé bīng* (Mentholum) 50g into *Jīn Huáng Sǎn* (金黄散) and grind them together into a smooth and even powder.

For terrible pain or itchiness, add 10% powdered *bái liǎn* (Radix Ampelopsis).

For dusky or dull-colored complexion, add 10% powdered *dāng guī* (Radix Angelicae Sinensis).

For excessive sebum secretion, add 10% powdered *bái xiān pí* (Cortex Dictamni) and 5% podwered *liú huáng* (Sulfur).

Mix 15-25g *Jīn Huáng Sǎn* (金黄散) into a pasty substance. Then apply uniformly to the affected area and leave for 30 minutes. Repeat this procedure every evening. If the paste feels slightly dry, add water to keep it moist.[16]

Huang Lin created an empirical formula *Rú Yì Xǐ Jì* (如意洗剂) to treat 135 cases of acne. The medicinals include: *rú yì cǎo* (Lantana camara), *gān shè xiāng* (dry Moschus), *dà yè ān* (Eucalyptus robusta Sm), *jīn yín huā* (Flos Lonicerae Japonicae), and *bò hé* (Herba Menthae). Decoct and drain the liquid to make a liniment.

He also created *Lián Shí Sǎn* (连石散) by grinding *huáng lián* (Rhizoma Coptidis), *lú gān shí* (Galamina), *bò hé* (Herba Menthae), *bīng piàn* (Borneolum Syntheticum), and *mì tuó sēng* (Lithargyrum) into powder. Both medicinal powders may be blended together.

Pour the *Rú Yì Xǐ Jì* (如意洗剂) into the palm and apply to the affected areas for about 1 minute until it begins to foam. Then wash off with warm water and dry the area. Then mix *Lián Shí Sǎn* (连石散) with water to make a paste and apply to the affected areas and let dry. Apply twice a day, in the morning and evening.[17]

Of the 135 cases, 88 cases fully recovered, 43 cases had some effect, and 4 cases showed no effect. The total effective rate was 97%.

Xu Ping-ji treated 100 cases of acne with *Shuāng Bái Sǎn* (satis quantum) (双白散). Grind *bái zhǐ* (Radix Angelicae Dahuricae) and *bái fù zǐ* (Rhizoma Typhonii) into a fine powder, and mix with water with a proportion of 6:4 powder to water. Apply to the affected areas once every evening.

With this method, 71 of the 100 cases were considered cured.[18]

4) Topical Application

Cao Yi had treated 1,120 cases of acne with a liniment based on a Chinese medicinal formula which mainly employs *jiāng huáng* (Rhizoma Curcumae Longae). The prescription is made up of 2% volatile oil of *jiāng huáng* (Rhizoma Curcumae Longae), 5% extract of *dān shēn* (Radix et Rhizoma Salviae Miltiorrhizae), 2.5% extract of *dāng guī* (Radix Angelicae Sinensis), 1% mycelium of *chóng cǎo* (Cordyceps), 1% extract of *rén shēn* (Radix Ginseng) and *tiān má* (Rhizoma Gastrodiae), and depurated *lú huì* (Aloe) 1g. A massage liniment was prepared by mixing these different extracts with Tween-azone oil. Using a cotton swab, apply the liniment to the affected area and massaged the area for 1-5 minutes. Apply 2-3 times a day for 1 month as one course of treatment.

In 1,000 cases, there was a 99.8% rate of effectiveness. For 120 cases of cyst and nodule acne types, the rate of effectiveness was 94.2%.[19]

Huang He-qing treated 34 cases of acne using *Hé Shǒu Wū Kǔ Shēn Hé Jì* (何首乌苦参合剂). Treating a total of 24 cases, 14 cases fully recovered, 9 cases had some effect, and only 1 case had no effect.

Place the following herbs into a wide-mouth glass bottle: *kǔ shēn* (Radix Sophorae Flavescentis) 50g, *shēng hé shǒu wū* (Radix Polygoni multiflori) 50g, *dāng guī* (Radix Angelicae Sinensis) 50g, and *bái zhǐ* (Radix

Angelicae Dahuricae) 50g. Add white vinegar and tighten the cap. Place the bottle in a pot of water and heat for 1 hour. Wait until the next day to open the bottle. Then pour some of the liquid onto a cotton ball and apply to the affected area. Apply twice a day, once each morning and evening. Twenty days constitutes one course of treatment.[20]

(3) Integration of Internal Treatment and External Treatment

Peng Guo-ying treated 110 cases of acne, and received a 95.5% effective rate using a formula called *Xiāo Cuò Yǐn* (消痤饮).

Ingredients: *gān fú líng* (dry Poria), *yì yǐ rén* (Semen Coicis), *yì mǔ cǎo* (Herba Leonuri), *kǔ shēn* (Radix Sophorae Flavescentis), *pú gōng yīng* (Herba Taraxaci), *bái zhǐ* (Radix Angelicae Dahuricae), and *huáng bǎi* (Cortex Phellodendri Chinensis). One bag of herbs per day, decocted.

Also, add 1000ml of water to *Xiāo Cuò Yǐn* (消痤饮), *bái huā shé shé cǎo* (Herba Hedyotis Diffusae), and *huáng lián* (Rhizoma Coptidis). Decoct as a facial steam directed at the affected area, apply twice a day.[21]

Han Shu-qin developed a treatment for acne by combining his own formula, *Jiě Dú Huà Yū Tāng* (解毒化瘀汤) with the external use of *Qīng Rè Huà Yū Xiāo Chuāng Sǎn* (清热化瘀消疮散). The formula for internal use was *Jiě Dú Huà Yū Tāng* (解毒化瘀汤).

Ingredients: *jīn yín huā* (Flos Lonicerae Japonicae), *pú gōng yīng* (Herba Taraxaci), *zǐ cǎo* (Radix Arnebiae), *zǐ huā dì dīng* (Herba Violae), *yě jú huā* (Flos Chrysanthemi Indici), *xià kū cǎo* (Spica Prunellae), *chì sháo* (Radix Paeoniae Rubra), *mǔ dān pí* (Cortex Moutan), *é zhú* (Rhizoma Curcumae), *sān qī* (Radix et Rhizoma Notoginseng), *chuān xiōng* (Rhizoma Chuanxiong), *fáng fēng* (Radix Saposhnikoviae), *bái zhǐ* (Radix Angelicae Dahuricae), and *chán tuì* (Periostracum Cicadae).

He also created an external facial treatment with *Qīng Rè Huà Yū Xiāo Chuāng Sǎn* (清热化瘀消疮散).

Ingredients: *fáng fēng* (Radix Saposhnikoviae) 10g, *jīng jiè* (Herba

Schizonepetae) 10g, *zǐ cǎo* (Radix Arnebiae) 10g, *chì sháo* (Radix Paeoniae Rubra) 10g, *cāng zhú* (Rhizoma Atractylodis) 15g, *pú gōng yīng* (Herba Taraxaci) 15g, *dà huáng* (Radix et Rhizoma Rhei) 6g, and *zào jiǎo cì* (Spina Gleditsiae) 6g. All ingredients are ground into a fine powder.

The first herbal formula, *Jiě Dú Huà Yū Tāng* (解毒化瘀汤) should be taken as one bag per day. Take twice a day, once each morning and evening. The second formula, *Qīng Rè Huà Yū Xiāo Chuāng Sǎn* (清热化瘀消疮散) is made into a Chinese medicinal facial mask for topical application, used once every 7 days. One month constitutes one course of treatment.

Of the 209 cases, 125 cases (43%) were cured after one course, 79 cases (37.8%) were cured after two courses, 3 cases (0.43%) were cured after three courses, and 2 cases (0.96%) were cured after more than three courses. The total rate of efficacy was 100%. [22]

Liu Pei-hong used Chinese medicinals that clear heat, resolve toxins, cool the blood and drain dampness for internal use, and other Chinese medicinals as a facial mask for external use.

Preparation of Chinese medicinals for oral use: *jīn yín huā* (Flos Lonicerae Japonicae) 15g, *yě jú huā* (Flos Chrysanthemi Indici) 15g, *chì sháo* (Radix Paeoniae Rubra) 15g, *shēng yì yǐ rén* (raw Semen Coicis) 30g, *dāng guī* (Radix Angelicae Sinensis) 15g, *zǐ cǎo* (Radix Arnebiae) 10g, *kǔ shēn* (Radix Sophorae Flavescentis) 10g, *xià kū cǎo* (Spica Prunellae) 10g, *mǎ chǐ xiàn* (Herba Portulacae) 30g, *dān shēn* (Radix et Rhizoma Salviae Miltiorrhizae) 15g and *bái huā shé shé cǎo* (Herba Hedyotis Diffusae) 15g.

Also mix *yě jú huā* (Flos Chrysanthemi Indici), *huáng qín* (Radix Scutellariae), *huáng lián* (Rhizoma Coptidis), *pú gōng yīng* (Herba Taraxaci), *lián qiào* (Fructus Forsythiae), *dān shēn* (Radix et Rhizoma Salviae Miltiorrhizae), *xià kū cǎo* (Spica Prunellae), and *bái huā shé shé cǎo* (Herba Hedyotis Diffusae) in equal parts. Grind the medicinals into a fine powder. Take 20g of the powder and mix with *shēng shí gāo* (raw Gypsum Fibrosum) 200g and water to form a paste. Apply it onto the affected area, and remove the mask after 20 minutes, after the mask has solidified. Apply this mask once every week. For severe cases, twice a week is applicable.

Of the 60 cases treated for acne, the effective rate was 95%.[23]

Liu Hong-xia had treated 100 cases of acne. All cases had an effect, with 80 cases showing a complete cure. The main treatment includes modifications of *Jīn Yín Huā Tāng* (金银花汤).

Ingredients: *jīn yín huā* (Flos Lonicerae Japonicae), *chē qián cǎo* (Herba Plantaginis), *lián qiào* (Fructus Forsythiae), *huáng qín* (Radix Scutellariae), *zǐ cǎo* (Radix Arnebiae), *shēng huái huā* (raw Flos Sophorae), *méi guī huā* (Flos Rosae Rugosae), *fú líng* (Poria), *zhū líng* (Polyporus), *dāng guī* (Radix Angelicae Sinensis), *kǔ shēn* (Radix Sophorae Flavescentis), and *shēng yì yǐ rén* (raw Semen Coicis). Take one bag per day, two times per day.

Place the herbs in a gauze-like pouch, add 2 L water and decoct for 30 minutes. Then use the decoction to steam the face for 5 minutes, until the face begins to sweat slightly. Once the decoction cools to a lukewarm temperature, soak a towel with the decoction and apply to the face for 30 minutes. To be applied once each evening. Also, mix *Diān Dǎo Sǎn* (颠倒散) or *Xiāo Shī Sǎn* (消失散) with boiling water and apply to the affected area with a towel or compress.[24]

Shen Yong utilized an internal treatment by using a decocted formula called *Xiāo Cuò Líng* (消痤灵).

Ingredients: *shēng dì huáng* (Radix Rehmanniae), *dāng guī* (Radix Angelicae Sinensis), *mǔ dān pí* (Cortex Moutan), *shēng gān cǎo* (raw Radix et Rhizoma Glycyrrhizae), *tiān huā fěn* (Radix Trichosanthis), *xuán shēn* (Radix Scrophulariae), *sāng bái pí* (Cortex Mori), *pí pá yè* (Folium Eriobotryae), *bái zhǐ* (Radix Angelicae Dahuricae), *huáng qín* (Radix Scutellariae), *chì sháo* (Radix Paeoniae Rubra), and *huáng lián* (Rhizoma Coptidis).

The external treatment included the application of *bái guǒ rén* (Semen

Ginkgo) extract. The oral prescription was one bag of *Xiāo Cuò Líng* (消痤灵) per day. One bag should be decocted and taken twice a day, once each morning and evening.

To prepare *bái guǒ rén* (Semen Ginkgo) extract, pound *bái guǒ rén* (Semen Ginkgo) into pieces, soak in 300ml ethanol for 7 days, and filter out the liquid. The affected area should be cleaned with sulfur soap and warm water before application of the extract.

Of the 98 cases, 64 had fully recovered, 17 of them had some effect, and 4 cases had no effect. The cure rate was 65.31%, and the total effective rate was 95.92%.[25]

Yu Bin used modifications of an empirical formula, *Xiāo Cuò Tāng* (消痤汤).

Ingredients: *jīng jiè* (Herba Schizonepetae), *fáng fēng* (Radix Saposhnikoviae), *huáng qín* (Radix Scutellariae), *bái zhǐ* (Radix Angelicae Dahuricae), *sāng bái pí* (Cortex Mori), *jīn yín huā* (Flos Lonicerae Japonicae), *yě jú huā* (Flos Chrysanthemi Indici), *shēng dì huáng* (Radix Rehmanniae), *dān shēn* (Radix et Rhizoma Salviae Miltiorrhizae), *chì sháo* (Radix Paeoniae Rubra), and *mǔ dān pí* (Cortex Moutan), applied as an oral medication.

He also used the formula, *Fù Fāng Dà Huáng Dīng* (复方大黄酊), soaked with a 75% concentration of ethanol for one week. The liquid is applied externally to the affected areas.

The formula consists of the following medicinals: *shēng dà huáng* (raw Radix et Rhizoma Rhei), sublime *liú huáng* (Sulfur), *zào jiǎo cì* (Spina Gleditsiae), *bǎi bù* (Radix Stemonae), *huáng bǎi* (Cortex Phellodendri Chinensis), and *hóng huā* (Flos Carthami). *Xiāo Cuò Tāng* (消痤汤) should be also decocted with water. To be taken once daily. Furthermore, the formula *Fù Fāng Dà Huáng Dīng* (复方大黄酊) should be applied before bedtime and then washed off the next morning.

Of the 126 cases, only 6 cases showed no effect. The total effective rate was 95.22%. [26]

Yu Ya-tao used *Xiāo Fēng Săn* (消风散) and *Xiāo Cuò Miàn Mó* (消痤面膜) to treat 30 cases of acne. Of these cases, 18 cases were cured, 11 cases received some effect, and 1 case had no results. The total rate of effectiveness was 97%.

Xiāo Fēng Săn (消风散) was taken as an oral medicine. The ingredients include: *jīng jiè* (Herba Schizonepetae), *fáng fēng* (Radix Saposhnikoviae), *chán tuì* (Periostracum Cicadae), *niú bàng zǐ* (Fructus Arctii), *kǔ shēn* (Radix Sophorae Flavescentis), *cāng zhú* (Rhizoma Atractylodis), *shí gāo* (Gypsum Fibrosum), *zhī mǔ* (Rhizoma Anemarrhenae), *dāng guī* (Radix Angelicae Sinensis), *shēng dì huáng* (Radix Rehmanniae), *hú má* (Semen Sesami Nigrum), and *gān căo* (Radix et Rhizoma Glycyrrhizae).

Xiāo Cuò Miàn Mó (消痤面膜) was applied externally. Ingredients: *jīn yín huā* (Flos Lonicerae Japonicae), *lián qiào* (Fructus Forsythiae), *yě jú huā* (Flos Chrysanthemi Indici), *dà huáng* (Radix et Rhizoma Rhei), and *bái zhǐ* (Radix Angelicae Dahuricae). Take equal parts of the above herbs and grind them into a fine powder (such that it filters through 120 mesh sieve). Mix 20g of *Xiāo Cuò Miàn Mó* (消痤面膜) powder and *shēng shí gāo* (raw Gypsum Fibrosum) 20g with purified water to make a paste-like substance for a facial mask. With the patient lying down, clean and massage the face using a massage cream. Then remove the cream and apply the mask uniformly, starting from the root of the nose.[27]

(4) Additional Treatment Modalities

1) Point Therapy

Cao Wei-min used three-edged needles to prick 1-2 *ashi* points that displayed brown lesions on the back and on the chest. He utilized the bleeding technique by cupping the pricked points to drain 1-2ml of blood. This technique should be performed once every other day, with ten treatments constituting one course of treatment. Allow 3-4 days between each course of treatment. A total of 396 acne cases were treated.

After 1-3 courses, the total effective effective rate was 100%, and the total recovery rate was 90.4%.[28]

Duan Xin-ping applied the bleeding technique to acupuncture points BL 13 (*fèi shù*), BL 17 (*gé shù*), BL 20 (*pí shù*), BL 15 (*xīn shù*), and BL 21 (*wèi shù*) bilaterally. He divided patients into two groups and alternated acupuncture points between each group. Quickly prick the points with a sterile three-edged needle and apply the cupping technique for 10 minutes. 48 cases were treated with this method once every other day, ten treatments constituting one course of treatment.

The recovery rate was 52%, and the total effective rate was 96%.[29]

You Fu-shan selected *ashi* points on the back, and particularly points DU 14 (*dà zhuī*), DU 1 (*cháng qiáng*), and BL 13 (*fèi shù*). All points were treated with a fire needling to a depth of 0.5-1.0 *cun*. Needles are immediately withdrawn and cupped for 15 minutes. This technique should be performed once every two days, with 10 treatments constituting one course of treatment.

Of the 107 cases, all subjects improved to some degree. The total recovery rate was 91.6%.[30]

Ren You-hong used the fire needling technique combined with cupping and bleeding on acupuncture points on the back. Of the 58 acne cases, 42 cases were cured, 12 cases improved, and 4 cases had no effect. The overall effective rate was 93%.

These three techniques seem to have a remarkable effect when used together:

A. Bleeding and cupping method: With the patient lying face down, clean DU 14, BL 13, BL 17, BL 20, BL 23 bilaterally with the standard antiseptic protocol. Then use a plum-blossom (seven-star) needle to tap until the skin becomes flushed, red, and slightly bleeding. Then cup the areas for 5-10 minutes to draw out about 1-3ml blood.

B. Fire needling technique: With the patient lying face down, clean the acupuncture points with the standard antiseptic protocol. Hold the acupuncture needle above a burning flame until the needle becomes red and slightly white. Immediately prick into the center of the acne and then quickly withdraw the needle. Extract the pus or blood with cotton. For cystic or nodule types, this technique is not necessary. Instead, use a three-edged needle to prick around the acne and then extract the pus and/or blood in the same manner.

It is best to use a fine needle (1.4 mm diameter) when performing the fire needling technique on the face. The proper depth is such that the needle tip should penetrate through the affected tissue (acne) but not so deep as to penetrate the normal tissues. The above treatment should be done once a week. Four to six treatments constitute one course of treatment.[31]

2) Ear Acupuncture Points Treatment

Xuan Jiong-hua treated acne by needling 7-9 ear acupuncture points. The ear points were lung, liver, kidney, stomach, esophagus, large Intestine, endocrine, subcortex, cheek, and eye. He then split 2 mm mung beans and used adhesive fabric to paste them onto the ear. This is to be done on the left or right ear alternatively, once every five days. The patient should press on these areas for 1-2 minutes, several times a day. He utilized the above method to treat 100 cases of acne with an overall effectiveness of 96%.[32]

Chen Su-hua utilized the bleeding technique with three-edged needles to prick the ear apex of both ears. He also pricked the vein on the back of the ear and squeezed at least ten drops of blood from each side. For severe inflammation, 5% alficetin liquid medicine was also applied. Of the 192 cases of acne, 131 cases fully recovered (68%). The overall rate of effectiveness was 90%.[33]

Chen Ping selected ear acupuncture points such as *shenmen*, endocrine, subcortex, adrenal gland, lung, stomach, and large intestine. After proper cleaning, *wáng bù liú xíng* (Semen Vaccariae) is placed onto the center of an adhesive fabric (0.7 × 0.7cm in size) and affixed onto the selected ear points. The adhesive should be changed 3-4 times per day. With each new adhesive, the patient should press them ten times. The adhesive is placed on only one ear, alternating ears each time. Treatment should be applied once every 3 days, with ten treatments constituting one course of treatment.

Of the 92 cases, the recovery cure rate was 77.2% and the total effective rate was 90.2%.[34]

3) Combining Body Acupuncture with Ear Acupoints

Wang Li-ping employed the bleeding technique using three-edged needles on ear points cheek, forehead, and ear apex. She also placed adhesives with *wáng bù liú xíng* (Semen Vaccariae) onto ear points lung, large intestine, heart, spleen, endocrine, and adrenal gland. The patient is instructed to press them several times each day. Additionally, she pricked to bleed BL 15, BL 13, BL 17, BL 25 and other local reactive points, using a three-edged needle. Cupping was applied to remove a few drops of blood. This method should be performed once every 3 days, with 5 treatments constituting one course of treatment. Allow 3 days between each course of treatment.

Among the 180 cases, 144 cases fully recovered. The overall rate of effectiveness was 98.9%.[35]

Jiang Fang-wu utilized the bleeding technique on the ear helix. He first cleaned them thoroughly and then used a small knife to create 10-15 incisions, 0.3 cm in length. They were bled until 10-15 droplets of blood appeared, then pressed with a cotton ball to stop the bleeding. He also drew 4ml of blood from the brachial veins and quickly re-injected the blood back into ST 36 (*zú sān lǐ*), with equal amounts of blood into each leg. Both techniques were applied in the same treatment session, with treatments performed once every 2 weeks. Six treatments constituted one course of treatment.

Of the 86 cases of acne treated, the overall rate of effectiveness was 93%.[36]

4) Combining Chinese Medicinals and Acupuncture

Wang Xiao-tian method included the needling of ear points lung, stomach, endocrine, subcortex and *shenmen*, based on the presenting syndrome. He then applied *wáng bù liú xíng* (Semen Vaccariae) on the acupoints and instructed the patient to press them 3-4 times per day, at least 30 times each time. The *wáng bù liú xíng* (Semen Vaccariae) adhesive was changed on a daily basis. Seven days constituted one course of treatment. He also prescribed modifications of *Shēng Huā Yǐn* (生花饮) which included: *huáng bǎi* (Cortex Phellodendri Chinensis), *huáng qín* (Radix Scutellariae), *lián qiào* (Fructus Forsythiae), *yě jú huā* (Flos Chrysanthemi Indici), *shān zhā* (Fructus Crataegi), *jī nèi jīn* (Endothelium Corneum Gigeriae Galli), *sāng bái pí* (Cortex Mori), *pí pá yè* (Folium Eriobotryae), *páo jiǎ* (quick-fried Squama Manis), and *chuān xiōng* (Rhizoma Chuanxiong). Decoct in water once per day; to be taken once each morning and evening. Three weeks constituted one course of treatment.

Of the 204 acne cases, the recovery rate was 46.1% and total effective rate was 100%.[37]

Xu Jia used a combination of acupuncture, plum-blossom needling, bloodletting of ear acupoints, and Chinese herbal medicine to treat 80 cases of acne. There was also a control group of 80 patients who were treated only with Chinese medicine. After 2-3 courses of treatment, there was a statistical significance ($p<0.01$) between the experimental group's rate of effectiveness (97.5%) as compared to the control (67.5%).

A. Acupuncture Points: LI 4 (*hé gǔ*), DU 14, BL 13, ST 36.

➢ For damp heat, add LI 11 (*qǔ chí*) and ST 44 (*nèi tíng*).

➢ For blood stasis and phlegm congestion, add LR 3 (*tài chōng*) and ST 40 (*fēng lóng*).

Prick the perimeter of the affected area with 1 inch needles at a 15 degree angle. The distance between the two needles should be 0.5 inch. Apply the reducing technique, and retain the needles for 30 minutes. Ten treatments constitute one course of treatment; 2-3 courses of treatment were applied.

B. Plum-blossom needling: Tap the affected area with a plum-blossom needle and let it bleed slightly. Squeeze out blood and pus and then apply an appropriate amount of *An Er Idione* (iodine skin disinfectant). The patient should wash it off after 4-5 hours.

C. Bloodletting ear points: Rub the ear for 1 minute to increase blood flow to the ear. Then make a 1 mm incision and remove 10 drops of blood. Select two points each time, including points ear apex, endocrine, lung, and large intestine. Treat both ears, alternating points each treatment.

D. Chinese medicinal selection based on pattern differentiation

Damp-heat in the lung and stomach: Select *pí pá yè* (Folium Eriobotryae) 10g, *huáng qín* (Radix Scutellariae) 10g, *shēng shān zhī* (raw Fructus Gardeniae) 10g, *shēng dì* (Radix Rehmanniae) 10g, *huáng lián* (Rhizoma Coptidis) 6g, *shēng dà huáng* (raw Radix et Rhizoma Rhei) 3g, *yīn chén* (Herba Artemisiae Scopariae) 15g, and *bái huā shé shé cǎo* (Herba Hedyotis Diffusae) 30g.

Blood stasis and phlegm congestion: Select *táo rén* (Semen Persicae) 10g, *dāng guī* (Radix Angelicae Sinensis) 10g, *zhì bàn xià* (Rhizoma Pinelliae Praeparatum) 10g, *zhè bèi mǔ* (Bulbus Fritillariae Thunbergii) 10g, *hóng huā* (Flos Carthami) 10g, *chuān xiōng* (Rhizoma Chuanxiong) 6g, *chén pí* (Pericarpium Citri Reticulatae) 6g, *pú gōng yīng* (Herba Taraxaci) 15g, and *jīn yín huā* (Flos Lonicerae Japonicae) 10g.

Note: The control group was treated only with Chinese herbal medicine, as above.

Experimental Studies

1. RESEARCH ON THE EFFICACY OF SINGLE CHINESE MEDICINALS

Huang Tian chose 48 Chinese herbs and researched their ability to inhibit propionibacterium acne on the superficial layers of the skin.

Results showed that *dān shēn* (Radix et Rhizoma Salviae Miltiorrhizae), *lián qiào* (Fructus Forsythiae), *hŭ zhàng* (Rhizoma Polygoni Cuspidati), *huáng băi* (Cortex Phellodendri Chinensis), *shān dòu gēn* (Radix et Rhizoma Sophorae Tonkinensis), *dà huáng* (Radix et Rhizoma Rhei), *huáng lián* (Rhizoma Coptidis), and *yīn chén hāo* (Herba Artemisiae Scopariae) showed a high reactivity to propionibacterium acnes.

Huáng qín (Radix Scutellariae), *lóng dăn căo* (Radix Gentianae), *dà qīng yè* (Folium Isatidis), *jīn yín huā* (Flos Lonicerae Japonicae), *dì yú* (Radix Sanguisorbae), *băi bù* (Radix Stemonae), *qín pí* (Cortex Fraxini), *jiāo mù* (Zanthoxylum Bungeanum Mazim), *dāng guī* (Radix Angelicae Sinensis), *chuān xiōng* (Rhizoma Chuanxiong), *chóng lóu* (Rhizoma Paridis), and *zĭ huā dì dīng* (Herba Violae) displayed medium reactivity.

Of these 20 herbs, 15 clear heat, and 3 invigorate blood.[39]

Xia Ming-jing studied bacteriostasis and Chinese herbal medicine using the agar diffusion test. He found the major chemical constituents of *dà huáng* (Radix et Rhizoma Rhei), *dān shēn* (Radix et Rhizoma Salviae Miltiorrhizae), *huáng qín* (Radix Scutellariae) to be emodin, berberine, tanshinone, and baicalin, which actually showed a moderate inhibitory effect on propionibacterium acnes. Its inhibitory factor is 10-20 mm, which is superior to arilin.[40]

Wu Xiao-hong researched the herbs in the formula *Shé Dān Fāng* (蛇丹方).

These include *bái huā shé shé cǎo* (Herba Hedyotis Diffusae), *dān shēn* (Radix et Rhizoma Salviae Miltiorrhizae), *huáng qín* (Radix Scutellariae), *xià kū cǎo* (Spica Prunellae), *zhì dà huáng* (prepared Radix et Rhizoma Rhei), *lián qiào* (Fructus Forsythiae), *pú gōng yīng* (Herba Taraxaci), *é zhú* (Rhizoma Curcumae), *shēng shān zhā* (raw Fructus Crataegi), *yì mǔ cǎo* (Herba Leonuri), and *bái jí lí* (Fructus Tribuli).

Each herb displayed a bacteriostatic effect on propionibacterium types of acnes to varying degrees. That is, all herbs in this formula displayed some ability to inhibit the growth of bacteria. *Zhì dà huáng* (prepared Radix et Rhizoma Rhei) shows the strongest bacteriostatic effect, which is also equivalent to medicines such as minocycline and clindamycin. The herbs *dān shēn* (Radix et Rhizoma Salviae Miltiorrhizae), *huáng qín* (Radix Scutellariae), and *pú gōng yīng* (Herba Taraxaci), showed a secondary level of strength, however they showed better effects than the western medications erythromycin, alpen, tetracycline, and cidomycin. *Lián qiào* (Fructus Forsythiae), *é zhú* (Rhizoma Curcumae, *shēng shān zhā* (raw Fructus Crataegi), *xià kū cǎo* (Spica Prunellae), *bái jí lí* (Fructus Tribuli), *bái huā shé shé cǎo* (Herba Hedyotis Diffusae), and *yì mǔ cǎo* (Herba Leonuri) displayed a slightly weaker bacteriostatic effect.[41]

2. Research on Bacteriostatic Chinese Medicinal Formulas

Xuan Guo-wei conducted experiments on the superficial layer of the skin to research the bacteriostatic effect of *Xiāo Cuò Líng Dīng* (消痤灵酊).

The formula contains: *dān shēn* (Radix et Rhizoma Salviae Miltiorrhizae), *lián qiào* (Fructus Forsythiae), *chuān xīn lián* (Herba Andrographis), *bái zhǐ* (Radix Angelicae Dahuricae), *huáng qí* (Radix Astragali), and *gān cǎo* (Radix et Rhizoma Glycyrrhizae).

Results confirmed that *Xiāo Cuò Líng Dīng* shows good bacteriostatic effect on propionibacterium acne, staphylococcus aureus, staphylococcus albus, and bacillus coli.

Ding Li-zhong researched the therapeutic effect of *Sān Bái Yǐn* (三白饮) on rabbit acne models, as well as its bacteriostasis effect in vitro. *Sān Bái Yǐn* consisted of *bái jiāng cán* (Bombyx Batryticatus), *bái huā shé shé cǎo* (Herba Hedyotis Diffusae), *bái zhǐ* (Radix Angelicae Dahuricae), *lián qiào* (Fructus Forsythiae), etc. Results showed that *Sān Bái Yǐn* displays bacteriostatic effects in vitro on propionibacterium acnes, staphylococcus aureus, malassezia furfur, and especially propionibacterium acnes. [43]

Zhang Fei studied bacteriostasis on the superficial areas of the skin using *Jīn Jú Xiāng Jiān Jì* (金菊香煎剂) to treat propionibacterium acne. He found that no colonies appeared in an anaerobic culture where *Jīn Jú Xiāng Jiān Jì* (金菊香煎剂) was applied.

The herbs in *Jīn Jú Xiāng Jiān Jì* (金菊香煎剂) are: *jīn yín huā* (Flos Lonicerae Japonicae), *yě jú huā* (Flos Chrysanthemi Indici), *huáng qín* (Radix Scutellariae), *zhī zǐ* (Fructus Gardeniae), *sāng bái pí* (Cortex Mori), *dì gǔ pí* (Cortex Lycii), *quán guā lóu* (Fructus Trichosanthis), *shú dà huáng* (prepared Radix et Rhizoma Rhei), *xiāng fù* (Rhizoma Cyperi), and *yì mǔ cǎo* (Herba Leonuri). [44]

Shen Dong researched the effects of the formula *Fù Fāng Shé Cǎo Tāng* (复方蛇草汤). The ingredients of this formula include *bái huā shé shé cǎo* (Herba Hedyotis Diffusae), *dān shēn* (Radix et Rhizoma Salviae Miltiorrhizae), *yì mǔ cǎo* (Herba Leonuri), *huáng qín* (Radix Scutellariae), *lóng dǎn cǎo* (Radix Gentianae), *xià kū cǎo* (Spica Prunellae), *cāng zhú* (Rhizoma Atractylodis), *bái jí lí* (Fructus Tribuli), *lián qiào* (Fructus Forsythiae), and *shēng shí gāo* (raw Gypsum Fibrosum). The decoction and distilled water were separately applied to propionibacterium acnes. Results showed that *Fù Fāng Shé Cǎo Tāng* (复方蛇草汤) decoction displayed high reactivity with propionibacterium acnes in every case. [45]

3. Research on Chinese Medicinals and Sebum Secretion

Feng Yong-fang researched the effect of herbal medicine on hamster models. He administered the experimental group *Cuò Chuāng Gāo* (痤疮膏), which contains: *dà huáng* (Radix et Rhizoma Rhei), *kǔ shēn* (Radix Sophorae Flavescentis), *huáng lián* (Rhizoma Coptidis), *bái zhǐ* (Radix Angelicae Dahuricae), *jiāng cán* (Bombyx Batryticatus), *bái jí* (Rhizoma Bletillae), *táo rén* (Semen Persicae), and *fú líng* (Poria). An Spironolactone group was used as a control. Results indicated that *Cuò Chuāng Gāo* had similar effects to the antagonist spironolactone and could effectively inhibit hyperplasia of sebaceous glands in hamsters.[46]

Li Bin of Yueyang hospital discovered that *Qīng Fèi Qū Zhī Fāng* (清肺祛脂方) could make a significant contribution to the treatment of acne by inhibiting sebum secretions. The blood serum free fatty acids significantly decreased after the use of this herbal formula. The function of *Qīng Fèi Qū Zhī Fāng* (清肺祛脂方) is to clear the lung and cool blood.[47]

Wang Wu-qing researched the effects of the Chinese herbal medicine *Cuò Chuāng Yǐn* (痤疮饮) on the sebum secretion rate of acne patients. To measure the effect of this herbal formula on the sebum secretion rate he used the Samuelson system, "nine degree classification"(*Jiu Du Fen Ji Fa*), and the Modified Zhou Family Direct Weight Method (*Zhou Shi Zhi Jie Cheng Zhong Fa*). The herbs in *Cuò Chuāng Yǐn* (痤疮饮) include: *jīn yín huā* (Flos Lonicerae Japonicae), *pú gōng yīng* (Herba Taraxaci), *zǐ huā dì dīng* (Herba Violae), *shēng dì huáng* (Radix Rehmanniae), and *huáng bǎi* (Cortex Phellodendri Chinensis). Results indicated that *Cuò Chuāng Yǐn* (痤疮饮) effectively lowers sebum secretion rates.[48]

Ding Li-zhong performed research on the formula *Sān Bái Yǐn* (三白饮). It displays the ability to inhibit keratosis, sebum secretions, keratosis at the hair follicle, and fatty acid secretions. It also decreases capillary permeability and thus inhibits acute exudation and inflammation while also enhancing the phagocytic function of the endothelial system.[43]

4. Dān Shēn (Radix et Rhizoma Salviae Miltiorrhizae) Acne Treatment

A chemical component called tanshinone can be extracted from *dān shēn* (Radix et Rhizoma Salviae Miltiorrhizae). According to medical literature, this extract mimics hormonal function in that it is anti-androgenic, anti-bacterial, and anti-inflammatory, with the additional function of regulating immune function.[49]

REFERENCES

[1] Li Zheng. Observation on Curative Effect of Treating 136 Cases of Acne Vulgaris According to Pattern Differentiation. (辨证分型治疗寻常性痤疮136例疗效观察). *The Chinese Journal of Dermatovenereology* (中国皮肤性病学杂志). 1997, 11(5): 294.

[2] Zhang Hong-ya, Liu Zheng, Ge Ming, et al. Treating 196 Cases of Acne According to Pattern Differentiation. (辨证论治痤疮196例). *Journal of Anhui Traditional Chinese Medical College* (安徽中医学院学报). 1997,16(4) : 29-30.

[3] Feng Jian-hua. Understanding the Treatment Acne Based on Pattern Differentiation. (痤疮辨治体会). *Shandong Journal of Traditional Chinese Medicine* (山东中医杂志). 2005, (5): 281-282.

[4] Xiong Ya-li. Using Modifications of *Yu Nu Jian* to Treat 120 Cases of Common Acne. (玉女煎加减治疗寻常痤疮120例). *Hunan Journal of Traditional Chinese Medicine* (湖南中医杂志). 1998, 14 (3): 65.

[5] Han Yong-sheng, Han Ping. Treating 20 Cases of Acne with Modifications of *Pi Pa Qing Fei Yin* (枇杷清肺饮加减治疗痤疮20例). *Xinjiang Journal of Traditional Chinese Medicine* (新疆中医药). 1998, 16 (1) : 27.

[6] Xu Xin. Treating 50 cases of Acne on the Face with Additions of *Pu Ji Xiao Du Yin* (普济消毒饮加味治疗面部痤疮50例). *Journal of Henan University of Chinese Medicine* (河南中医学院学报). 2005, 7(4): 119.

[7] Yang Wen-xin, Zhang Jian. Treating 712 Cases of Acne With *Yun Pi San Jie Tang* (运脾散结汤治疗痤疮712例). *Journal of Sichuan Traditional Chinese Medicine* (四川中医). 2005, (1): 73.

[8] Liang Shang-cai. Treating 400 Cases of Common Acne with *Fen Ci Jian* (粉刺煎治疗寻常痤疮400例). *Jilin Journal of Traditional Chinese Medicine* (吉林中医药). 1998,18 (2) : 42

[9] Yang En-pin. Clinical Analysis on the Treatment of 120 Cases of Common Facial Acne with *Cuo Chuang Qiang Xiao Yin* (痤疮清消饮治疗面部寻常痤疮102例临床分析). *Yunnan Journal of Traditional Chinese Medicine and Materia Medica* (云南中医中药杂志). 1997, 18 (1): 24..

[10] Yang Ying-cheng, Li Ying-feng. Treating 130 Cases of Acne with Chinese Facial Mask (中药倒模治疗痤疮130例). *Journal of External Therapy of Traditional Chinese Medicine* (中医外治杂志). 1996, (5): 17.

[11] Yan Lu-juan & Zhao jian. Treating 36 Cases of Facial Acne with Chinese Facial Mask (中药倒模治疗面部痤疮36例). *Jilin Journal of Traditional Chinese Medicine* (吉林中医药). 1996, (4): 25.

[12] Shi Ping. Clinical Observations of Treating Common Facial Acne with Chinese Medicine Facial Mask (中药面膜治疗面部寻常痤疮临床观察). *Chinese Journal for Clinicians* (中国临床医生). 2005, (1): 53.

[13] Ren Zhi-min, Zhao Li-jie. Clinical Observations of Treating 500 Cases of Common Acne with Method of Fumigating and Washing (熏洗法治疗寻常痤疮500例临床观察). *Chinese Journal of Traditional Medical Science and Technology* (中国中医药科技). 1998, 5 (1): 59.

[14] Wang Xiao-hong. Treating 60 Cases of Acne with Method of Fumigating and Washing (中药熏洗法治疗痤疮60例). *Journal of Nanjing University of Traditional Chinese Medicine University* (南京中医药大学学报). 1997, 13 (5): 309.

[15] Shu Gui-tian. Treating 17 Cases of Acne with the Application of *Tu Si Zi* (菟丝子汁外用治疗痤疮17例). *Zhejiang Journal of Traditional Chinese Medicine* (浙江中医杂志). 1996, 31 (4): 179.

[16] Zhang Lei, Wang Wei. Treating 500 Cases of Common Acne with Additions of *Jin Huang San* (金黄散加味调制治疗寻常性痤疮). *Journal of External Therapy of Traditional Chinese Medicine* (中医外治杂志). 1998, 7 (1) : 40.

[17] Huang Lin. Clinical Observations of Curative Effect of Treating 135 Cases of Acne with *Ru Yi Lotion* (如意洗剂外治痤疮135例疗效观察). *New Journal of Traditional Chinese Medicine* (新中医). 1997, 29 (7): 42.

[18] Xu Ping-ji. Treating Acne 100 Cases with *Shuang Bai San* (双白散治疗痤疮100例). *Journal of External Treatment of Chines Medicine* (中医外治杂志). 1995, 4 (6): 32.

[19] Cao Yi. Clinical Observations on the Efficacy of *Jiang Huang's* Chinese Medicine Preparation (姜黄为主的复方中药制剂治疗痤疮的疗效观察). *Chinese Journal of Dermatology* (中华皮肤科杂志), 1996, (4) : 280.

[20] Huang He-qing, Huang Jun, Du Zhi-gang. Applying *Ku Shen He Shou Wu* Mixture to Treat Acne (苦参何首乌合剂外擦治疗痤疮). *Zhejiang Journal of Traditional Chinese Medicine* (浙江中医杂志). 1997, 32 (5): 213.

[21] Peng Guo-ying. Treating 110 Cases of Acne with External and Internal Treatment (内外兼治痤疮110例). *Henan Traditional Chinese Medicine* (河南中医). 1998, 18 (1): 52.

[22] Han Shu-qin, Zhang Dong-mei. Clinical Observations on the Efficacy of Treating 209 Acne Cases with by Relieving toxins and Transforming Stasis (特效解毒化瘀法治疗痤疮209例临床疗效观察). *Hebei Journal of Traditional Chinese Medicine* (河北中医). 1997, 19 (6): 11~13.

[23] Liu Pei-hong, Shu You-lian. Clinical Observations of Oral Chinese Herbal Combined with Chinese Facial Mask for Treating Common Acne. (中药内服配合中药倒膜外用治疗寻常痤疮临床观察). *Chinese Archives of Traditional Chinese Medicine* (中医药学刊). 2005, (8): 23.

[24] Liu Hong-xia. Treating 100 Cases of Acne with *Jin Yin Hua Tāng* (A Self- Composed Formula) (自拟金银花汤治疗痤疮100例). *Fujian Journal of Traditional Chinese Medicine* (福建中医药). 1996, (1): 28.

[25] Shen Yong. Treating 98 Cases of Acne with *Xiao Cuo Ling Tang* (消痤灵汤治疗痤疮98例).

Chinese Journal of Integrated Traditional and Western Medicine (中国中西医结合杂志). 1998,8 (6): 379~380.

[26] Yu Bin. Treating 126 Acne Cases with Oral Administration of *Xiao Cuo Tang* and The Topical Application of *Da Huang Ding* (内服消痤汤外擦大黄酊治疗痤疮126例). *Hunan Journal of Traditional Chinese Medicine* (湖南中医杂志). 1998, 14 (4): 40.

[27] Yu Ya-tao, Tian Shu-ying. Treating 30 Cases of Acne with *Xiao Feng San* Used As *Xiao Cuo Mian Mo* (消风散外用消痤面膜治疗痤疮30例). *Liaoning Journal of Traditional Chinese Medicine* (辽宁中医杂志) 2005, (6): 547.

[28] Cao Wei-min. Clinical Observations of Using Sharp Needles and Cupping to Treat 396 Cases of Acne (锋针配合火罐治疗痤疮396例疗效观察). *Chinese Acupuncture & Moxibustion* (中国针灸). 1995, 15 (5): 13.

[29] Duan Xin-ping. Using the Pricking Method with Three-edged Needles and Cupping to Treat 48 Cases of Facial Acne (三棱针挑刺加拔罐治疗面部粉刺48例). *Acupuncture Research* (针刺研究). 1998, 23 (3): 225.

[30] You Fu-shan. Treating Acne with Fire Needling Technique (火针刺治疗痤疮). *Journal of Clinical Acupuncture and Moxibustion* (针灸临床杂志). 1996, 12 (1): 31.

[31] Ren You-hong, Zhang Wen-ping, Chen Zhu-bi. Using Fire Needling Combined with Bloodletting, and Cupping to Treat 58 Cases of Acne (火针配合刺络拔罐治疗痤疮58例). *Shanghai Journal of Acupuncture and Moxibustion* (上海针灸杂志). 2005 (4): 16-17.

[32] Xuan Jiong-hua. Pressing Ear Acupuncture Points to Treat 100 Cases of Acne (耳穴贴压治疗痤疮100例). *Chinese Acupuncture & Moxibustion* (中国针灸). 1995, 15 (6) : 4.

[33] Chen Su-hua, Tang Yang-hong. Treating 192 Cases of Acne with Bleeding on Ear Acupuncture Points (耳穴点刺放血治疗痤疮192例). *Shanghai Journal of Acupuncture and Moxibustion* (上海针灸杂志). 1998,17 (3) : 31.

[34] Chen Ping, Zhang Xiu-hua, Li Yan. Pressing Ear Acupuncture Points with *Wang Bu Liu Xing* to Treat 192 Cases of Acne (耳压王不留行籽治疗痤疮92例). *Chinese Journal of Traditional Medical Science and Technology* (中国中医药科技), 1997,4 (4): 242.

[35] Wang Li-ping, Liu Bao-lin. Treating 108 Cases of Acne Combining Ear Acupuncture and Body Acupuncture (耳针与体针结合治疗痤疮108例). *Journal of Clinical Acupuncture and Moxibustion* (针灸临床杂志). 1996, 12 (10): 23.

[36] Jiang Fang-wu. Treating 86 Cases of Acne by Bloodletting the Ear Helix and Injecting the Patient's Own Blood into His own Acupoints (耳轮放血配合自血穴注治疗痤疮86例). *Yunnan Journal of Traditional Chinese Medicine and Materia Medica* (云南中医中药杂志). 1997, 18 (1): 37.

[37] Wang Xiao-tian. Observations of Treating 204 Cases of Common Acne with Pressing Ear Acupuncture Points Combined with Chinese Herbal Medicine (耳穴贴压配合中药治疗寻常痤疮204例观察). *Chinese Acupuncture & Moxibustion* (中国针灸). 1996, 16 (4): 11.

[38] Xu Jia. Treating 204 Cases of Acne Combining of Acupuncture and Chinese Medicine (针药结合治疗痤疮80例). *Journal of Nanjing University of Traditional Chinese Medicine University* (南京中医药大学学报), 2005, 5(3): 190-191.

[39] Huang Tian, Kong Li-jun, Sun Ling et al. The Inhibitory Effect of 48 Kinds of Chinese

Medicines on Propionibacterium Acnes (48种中药对痤疮丙酸杆菌的抑制作用). *Chinese Journal of Dermatology* (中华皮肤科杂志). 1992, (5): 307.

[40] Xia Ming-jing, Cao Yi, Yang Jie, et al. The Inhibitory Effect of 22 Kinds of Chinese Medicines on Propionibacterium Acnes (22种抗菌消炎中药有效成分对痤疮丙酸杆菌的抑制作用[J]). *Chinese Journal of Dermatology* (中华皮肤科杂志). 2001, 12 (6): 435-436).

[41] Wu Xiao-hong, Liu Wa-li, Yu Yong. The Inhibitory Effect of *She Dan Fang* and Medicine on Propionibacterium Acnes (中药蛇丹方及其构成生药对痤疮丙酸杆菌的抑菌作用). *Chinese Journal of Dermatovenerology of Integrated Traditional and Western Medicine* (中国中西医结合皮肤性病学杂志). 2003, 2(4): 122-224.

[42] Xuan Guo-wei, Fan Rui-qiang, Yin Yu-zhen, et al. A Multiple Randomized Control Study on Treating Acne with Chinese Medicine *Xiao Cuo Ling* (中药消痤灵治疗痤疮的多中心随机对照研究). *Journal of Guangzhou Collegeof Traditional Chinese Medicine* (广州中医学院学报). 1995, (3): 6.

[43] Ding Li-zhong, Zhang Nan-fang, Wang Zhi-gang. Treating Experimental Acne with *San Bai Yin* (三白饮治疗实验性痤疮). *Chinese Journal of Hospital Pharmacy* (中国医院药学杂志). 2003, 23 (11): 681-682.

[44] Zhang Fei, Wang Ping, Zhang Zhi-li et al. Clinical Observations of Treating Common Acne on Female Patients with *Jin Ju Xiang* Decoction and the Detection of Testosterone in Blood Serum [J] (金菊香煎剂治疗女性寻常性痤疮临床观察及血清睾酮检测[J]). *The Chinese Journal of Dermatovenereology* (中国皮肤性病学杂志). 2001, (1): 48-49.

[45] Shen Dong, Xu Xian. A Clinical and Experimental Study on Treating Common Acne with *She Cao Tang* [J] (复方蛇草汤治疗寻常性痤疮的临床与实验研究[J]). *Journal of Clinical Dermatology* (临床皮肤科杂志). 2000, (4): 201-203.

[46] Feng Yong-fang, Zhu Lin-xue, Gao Jin, et al. A Study on *Cuo Chuang Gao* Resisting Hyperplasia of Glandulae Sebaceae Maculae of Golden Hamster [J]) (痤疮膏抗金黄地鼠皮脂腺斑增生的研究). *Journal of Hubei College of Traditional Chinese Medicine* (湖北中医学院学报). 2002, 4(2): 21.

[47] Li Bin, Geng Lin, Xu Wen-bin et. al. Influence of Clearing the Lung and Cooling the Blood on Seborhea Rate and Free Fatty Acids in Blood Serum of Common Acne Patients [J] (清肺凉血法对寻常痤疮患者皮脂溢出率和血清游离脂肪酸的影响[J]). *Chinese Journal of Clinical Rehabilitation* (中国临床康复). 2004, 8(20)：

[48] Wang Wu-qing, Chen Mei-hua, Du Xi-xian et al. Influence of *Cuo Chuang Yin* on the Sebum Excretion Rate of Common Acne Patients[J] (痤疮饮对寻常痤疮患者皮脂分泌率的影响[J]). *Fujian Journal of Traditional Chinese Medicine* (福建中医药). 2004, 35(4): 7-8.

[49] Qin Wan-zhang. *Study on Dermatosis*.(皮肤病研究) Shanghai: Shanghai Scientific & Technical Publishers, 1990.130.

Alopecia Areata

by

Fan Rui-qiang
Chief Physician & Professor of Chinese External Medicine

Chen Da-can
Chief Physician & Professor of Chinese External Medicine

Chen Xiu-yang, M.S.TCM
Attending Physician of Chinese External Medicine

Xuan Guo-wei
Chief Physician & Professor of Chinese External Medicine

Hu Dong-liu, M.S. TCM
Associate Chief Physician of Chinese External Medicine

072 Acne & Alopecia

Alopecia Areata

OVERVIEW	75
CHINESE MEDICAL ETIOLOGY AND PATHOMECHANISM	77
CHINESE MEDICAL TREATMENT	77
Pattern Differentiation and Treatment	77
Additional Treatment Modalities	86
1. Chinese Patent Medicine	86
2. Acupuncture and Moxibustion	87
3. External Applications	91
4. Simple Prescriptions and Empirical Formulas	93
PROGNOSIS	94
PREVENTIVE HEALTHCARE	95
Regulation of Emotional and Mental Health	95
Lifestyle Modification	95
Dietary Recommendation	96
CLINICAL EXPERIENCE OF RENOWNED PHYSICIANS	99
Empirical Formulas	99
1. Gù Shèn Shēng Fà Tāng (固肾生发汤) (Liang Jian-hui)	99
2. Bǔ Shèn Yǎng Xuè Tāng (补肾养血汤) (Liu Hui-min)	100
3. Shén Yìng Yǎng Zhēn Tāng (神应养真汤) (Cheng Zhen)	101
4. Gōu Qí Huáng Qí Tāng (枸杞黄芪汤) (Luo Yu-guo)	102
5. Shēng Fà Wán (生发丸) (Shi Guan-qing)	103
Selected Case Studies	103
1. Case Studies of Zhang Zhi-li: Liver, Kidney and Blood Deficiency	103
2. Case Studies of Dong Jian-hua: Liver and Kidney Yin Deficiency	105
3. Case Studies of Xuan Guo-wei: Qi and Yin Deficiency	107
Discussions	108
1. Deng Tie-tao on Pattern Differentiation and Treatment	108
2. Dong Jian-hua on Kidney and Blood Tonification	110
3. Lü Zhi-lian on Alopecia Areata with Deficiency Predominating	112

  4. Li Shu-tang on Draining Water, Dispelling Dampness, and Transforming Phlegm ········ 113
PERSPECTIVES OF INTEGRATIVE MEDICINE ········ 114
Challenges and Solutions ········ 114
  Challenge #1: How to Prevent Progression ········ 114
  Challenge #2: How to Treat Critical Alopecia ········ 115
  Challenge #3: How to Treat Pediatric Alopecia ········ 116
  Challenge #4: How to Reduce Recurrence ········ 117
Insight from Empirical Wisdom ········ 117
  1. Percussopunctation and TDP Equipment ········ 119
  2. External Application of Yì Fà B Tincture and Hormones ········ 119
Summary ········ 122
  1. Syndrome Differentiation and Pathogenesis ········ 123
  2. Alopecia and Comprehensive Therapies ········ 124
  3. Research on Various Alopecia Types ········ 127
  4. Combining Corticosteroids with Chinese Medicinals ········ 128
  5. Descriptive Reports and Clinical Research ········ 130
SELECTED QUOTES FROM CLASSICAL TEXTS ········ 131
MODERN RESEARCH ········ 136
Clinical Research ········ 136
  1. Pattern Differentiation and Corresponding Treatment ········ 136
  2. Specific Formulas ········ 138
  3. Acupuncture and Moxibustion ········ 146
Experimental Studies ········ 148
  1. Research on the Efficacy of Herbal Prescriptions ········ 148
  2. Research on the Efficacy of Herbal Prescriptions ········ 149
REFERENCES ········ 151

OVERVIEW

Alopecia areata is a condition of hair loss in which round patches appear suddenly. Its onset is abrupt, but it develops slowly and tends to recur. The clinical manifestations are hair loss in patches without signs of inflammation and other symptoms around the affected areas on the scalp. A severe progression of the disease can lead to alopecia totalis (total loss of scalp hair) or alopecia universalis (complete loss of body hair). It is estimated that the prevalence is 0.1% among the general population. While alopecia areata can develop at any age, most cases appear between 5-40 years of age. Young adults are the most commonly seen group in the clinic. In addition, the incidence of this condition is equal in both men and women. There are no predominant occurrences within certain geographic areas or seasons. Of all alopecia areata patients, nearly 30% develop alopecia universalis, while 95% of the patients display alopecia locally on the scalp.

In biomedicine, the cause of alopecia areata is still not completely understood. At present, immune dysfunction is considered the main reason for its onset, with correlations to psychological factors, vasomotor activity, genetics, endocrine disorders, and infection. Alopecia areata is regarded as an autoimmune disease, often precipitated and aggravated by psychological factors. It is usually caused by long-term anxiety, sorrow or grief. Outbreaks may also occur due to sudden panic or despair. Alopecia patients may display personality tendencies such that 41% of them are introverted with unstable personalities, and 70% suffer from sleeping problems such as insomnia, excessive dreaming, difficulty falling asleep, and early awakening. The pathogenesis may involve mental-emotional tension that leads to dysfunction of the autonomic nervous system, increased tonicity of the sympathetic nervous system, and constant contraction of blood vessels, all of which lead to impaired blood supply and cell hypofunction of the radix pili, causing alopecia areata. About 10%-20% of these cases show a genetic predisposition. People with congenital allergic constitutions also tend to have alopecia areata. It is most difficult to treat children with alopecia areata who have an inherited susceptibility for allergies.

Alopecia areata is clearly related to psychological factors as well. First, the primary goal of clinical treatment is to break the negative physiological and psychological cycle by providing emotional support to distressed patients dealing with psychological burdens, establishing their confidence for complete recovery, and to also explore the precipating factors. Patients with significant psychological issues may be prescribed sedatives or antidepressant medications. Secondly, therapies should be selectively combined to treat both the interior and exterior issues associated with alopecia areata. Oral dicysteine can replenish keratin, while oral thymic peptide and levamisole may adjust immune functions. Oral corticosteroids may be used in severe or widespread alopecia areata. However, due to the risk of serious side effects, such as hypertension or cataracts, they are used only occasionally or for shorter periods of time. Nevertheless, this medication can be used for severe cases to prevent progression into alopecia universalis or alopecia totalis. For external treatment, 2%-5% loniten, 0.02% chlormethine hydrochloride, and 0.1% anthralin ointment should be applied to the scalp. Meanwhile, triamcinolone acetonide, betamethasone, atropine and Vitamin E may be injected at local areas. Auxiliary therapies, such as cryotherapy with liquid nitrogen or carbon dioxide snow, photochemotherapy (PUVA), and physiotherapies such as massage, ultraviolet radiation, sound frequency electrotherapy, and wax therapy could be utilized as well.

Alopecia areata pertains to the notion of "glossy scalp wind"(*yóu fēng*, 油风) in Chinese medicine. It is also referred to as "ghost-licked head"(*guǐ tiǎn tóu*, 鬼舔头) and "ghost-shaved head"(*guǐ tì tóu*, 鬼剃头).

CHINESE MEDICAL ETIOLOGY AND PATHOMECHANISM

Alopecia areata results from improper diet, disharmony of the seven emotions, excessive strain, prolonged disease, serious disease, or congenital conditions. All of these factors create depletion in the *zang-fu* organs, qi and blood imbalances, weakened hair follicles, and malnourishment of the hair. The general pathogenesis is either deficiency or excess. Deficiency in alopecia areata refers to deficiencies of qi and blood, as well as of the liver and kidney. Excess is caused by an improper diet characterized by excessive spicy, hot or greasy foods, or by emotional depressions transforming into fire. These two factors can result in blood heat engendering wind or blood stasis in the hair follicles, which ultimately can bring about hair loss. Pathological changes in the hair are closely associated with the liver, spleen and kidney. The main syndromes of alopecia areata are blood heat engendering wind, dual deficiencies of qi and blood, liver depression and blood stasis, and insufficiency of the liver and kidney. It is important to recognize that insufficiency of the liver and kidney is more commonly seen in the clinic than the other syndromes. According to the basic theory of Chinese medicine, the liver stores blood, hair is the surplus of the blood, and the kidney stores essence. Therefore, insufficiency of the liver and kidney leads to essence and blood depletion, which deprives the hair of proper nourishment. This fundamental premise serves as the guiding principle in the clinical diagnosis and treatment of alopecia areata.

CHINESE MEDICAL TREATMENT

Pattern Differentiation and Treatment

The general treatment principle is to clear blood heat and dispel blood stasis for excess syndromes, and to tonify deficiency and consolidate essence in deficiency syndromes. When blood heat is cleared, the blood can circulate properly in the vessels. When blood stasis is dispelled, new blood can be generated. Therefore, both clearing blood heat and dispelling blood stasis can increase nutrient absorption and blood supply at the hair root. Also, hair growth can be promoted by tonifying deficiencies and consolidating essence. Since hair is the manifestation of the kidney, and the bloom of the kidney is in the hair, various symptoms and signs of kidney deficiency are commonly seen among alopecia areata patients. In addition to that, since the liver stores blood, and the liver and kidney are of the same source, it is also important to enrich both liver and kidney.

(1) Liver and Kidney Deficiency

【Syndrome Characteristics】

Long term alopecia, withered yellow or gray hair, extensive hair loss, loss of body hair, family history of alopecia, weak knees, vertigo, tinnitus, dizziness, seminal emission, insomnia, excessive dreaming, aversion to cold, and cold limbs. The tongue is pale with a thin or peeled coating, and the pulse is thready or deep.

【Treatment Principle】

Nourish liver and kidney, replenish essence to promote hair regrowth.

【Commonly Used Medicinals】

Gǒu qǐ zǐ (Fructus Lycii), *tù sī zǐ* (Semen Cuscutae), *dāng guī* (Radix Angelicae Sinensis), *nǚ zhēn zǐ* (Fructus Ligustri Lucidi), *niú xī* (Radix Achyranthis Bidentatae) and *shān zhū yú* (Fructus Corni) nourish liver and kidney. *Hé shǒu wū* (Radix Polygoni Multiflori), *hēi zhī ma* (Semen Sesami Nigrum) and *sāng jì shēng* (Herba Taxilli) replenish essence to promote hair growth.

【Representative Formula】

Modified *Qī Bǎo Měi Rán Dān* (七宝美髯丹).

【Ingredients】

制何首乌	zhì hé shǒu wū	15g	Radix Polygoni Multiflori Praeparata cum Succo Glycines Sotae
枸杞子	gǒu qǐ zǐ	15g	Fructus Lycii
菟丝子	tù sī zǐ	15g	Semen Cuscutae
当归	dāng guī	10g	Radix Angelicae Sinensis
牛膝	niú xī	12g	Radix Achyranthis Bidentatae
补骨脂	bǔ gǔ zhī	15g	Fructus Psoraleae
茯苓	fú líng	15g	Poria

Decoct in 500 ml of water until 100 ml of the decoction is left. Take warm, twice a day.

【Formula Analysis】

Zhì hé shǒu wū (Radix Polygoni Multiflori Praeparata cum Succo Glycines Sotae), *gǒu qǐ zǐ* (Fructus Lycii), and *niú xī* (Radix Achyranthis Bidentatae) tonify the kidney and replenish essence. *Tù sī zǐ* (Semen Cuscutae), *dāng guī* (Radix Angelicae Sinensis), and *bǔ gǔ zhī* (Fructus Psoraleae) tonify the kidney and nourish blood. *Fú líng* (Poria) fortifies the spleen, benefits qi, and prevents the other cloying herbs from impairing the stomach and spleen. This formula acts to nourish without causing stagnation.

【Modifications】

➢ For yang deficiency, add *yín yáng huò* (Herba Epimedii) 12g, and *bā jǐ tiān* (Radix Morindae Officinalis) 12g to tonify the kidney and invigorate yang.

➢ For predominant yin deficiency, add *mò hàn lián* (Herba Ecliptae) 12g, *zhī mǔ* (Rhizoma Anemarrhenae) 12g, *mǔ dān pí* (Cortex Moutan) 12g, and *bēng dà wǎn* (Herba Centellae) 12g to nourish liver and kidney yin, clear heat, and cool the blood.

➢ For blood stasis, add *cè bǎi yè* (Cacumen Platycladi) 12g, and *dān shēn* (Radix et Rhizoma Salviae Miltiorrhizae) 12g to cool the blood, invigorate blood, and dispel stasis.

➢ For insomnia and excessive dreaming, add *wǔ wèi zǐ* (Fructus Schisandrae Chinensis) 12g, *yì zhì rén* (Fructus Alpiniae Oxyphyllae) 12g, *hé huān pí* (Cortex Albiziae) 12g, and *suān zǎo rén* (Semen Ziziphi Spinosae) 12g to quiet the heart, calm the spirit, and eliminate restlessness.

➢ In cases of emotional problems, add *dài zhě shí* (Haematitum) 15g, and *yù jīn* (Radix Curcumae) 10g to eliminate restlessness, resolve constraint, and suppress hyperactive yang with heavy settling medicinals.

(2) Liver Constraint and Blood Stasis

【Syndrome Characteristics】

Other symptoms may have been present previous to the hair loss such as headache, stabbing pain on the scalp, and chest and rib-side pain. Patchy hair loss may appear, later developing into alopecia totalis. Other symptoms include nightmares, restlessness, irritability, chest distress and pain, hypochondriac distention, sighing, and insomnia. The tongue is dusky purple tongue or with stasis maculae and scant coating. The pulse is wiry or deep and choppy.

【Treatment Principle】

Course the liver and resolve constraint, invigorate blood, and resolve stasis.

【Commonly Used Medicinals】

To course the liver and resolve constraint, select *chái hú* (Radix Bupleuri), *sù xīn huā* (Flos Jasmini), and *yù jīn* (Radix Curcumae). To invigorate blood and resolve stasis, select *dān shēn* (Radix et Rhizoma Salviae Miltiorrhizae), *táo rén* (Semen Persicae), *hóng huā* (Flos Carthami), and *jī xuè téng* (Caulis Spatholobi).

【Representative Formula】

Modified *Xiāo Yáo Sǎn* (逍遥散) with *Táo Hóng Sì Wù Tāng* (桃红四物汤).

【Ingredients】

柴胡	chái hú	12g	Radix Bupleuri
白芍	bái sháo	20g	Radix Paeoniae Alba
茯苓	fú líng	15g	Poria
丹参	dān shēn	10g	Radix et Rhizoma Salviae Miltiorrhizae
赤芍	chì sháo	12g	Radix Paeoniae Rubra
当归	dāng guī	12g	Radix Angelicae Sinensis
熟地黄	shú dì huáng	30g	Radix Rehmanniae Praeparata
川芎	chuān xiōng	6g	Rhizoma Chuanxiong
桃仁	táo rén	9g	Semen Persicae
红花	hóng huā	9g	Flos Carthami
酸枣仁	suān zǎo rén	30g	Semen Ziziphi Spinosae
甘草	gān cǎo	6g	Radix et Rhizoma Glycyrrhizae

Decoct in 500 ml of water until 100 ml of the decoction is left. Take warm, twice daily.

【Formula Analysis】

Chái hú (Radix Bupleuri) courses the liver and resolves constraint to smooth the liver qi. It also serves as the chief medicinal in the formula. *Dāng guī* (Radix Angelicae Sinensis) acts to nourish and harmonize the blood with its sweet, acrid, bitter and warm nature. *Bái sháo* (Radix Paeoniae Alba) acts to nourish blood, astringe yin, and emolliate the liver with its sour, bitter, and mildly cold nature. *Dāng guī* (Radix Angelicae Sinensis) and *bái sháo* (Radix Paeoniae Alba) serve together as deputy medicinals. When blood is harmonized, the liver is harmonized; when the blood is sufficient, the liver becomes emolliated. Combined with *chái hú* (Radix Bupleuri), they together nourish the liver and promote its function. Since liver constraint impairs the spleen's ability to transform and transport, *fú líng* (Poria) and *gān cǎo* (Radix et Rhizoma Glycyrrhizae) fortify the spleen and benefit qi in order to promote generation of nutrient blood. Combined together, these medicinals course the liver to resolve constraint, nourish deficient blood, and strengthen the spleen.

They act to treat qi and blood simultaneously, while regulating the liver and nourishing blood. *Shú dì huáng* (Radix Rehmanniae Praeparata) enters the liver and kidney channels with its sweet flavor, and warm, thick and moist nature. It is regarded as a major blood-supplementing medicinal because of its ability to nourish yin and blood, supplement the kidney, and replenish essence. *Táo rén* (Semen Persicae) and *hóng huā* (Semen Persicae) act to break blood and resolve stasis.

【Modifications】

➢ For restless sleep, add *yè jiāo téng* (Caulis Polygoni Multiflori) 12g, *hé huān pí* (Cortex Albiziae) 12g, *zhēn zhū mǔ* (Concha Margaritiferae Usta) 30g, *cí shí* (Magnetitum) 30g, and *bǎi hé* (Bulbus Lilii) 9g to quiet the spirit with heavy settling herbs, nourish the heart, and eliminate restlessness.

➢ For liver constraint transforming into fire, add *mǔ dān pí* (Cortex Moutan) 9g and *zhī zǐ* (Fructus Gardeniae) 9g to clear heat and cool the blood.

➢ For serious liver constraint and qi stagnation with chest and rib-side pain, add *xiāng fù* (Rhizoma Cyperi) 9g, *chén pí* (Pericarpium Citri Reticulatae) 6g, and *yuán hú* (Rhizoma Corydalis) 12g to course the liver and resolve constraint to relieve pain.

(3) Blood Heat Engendering wind

【Syndrome Characteristics】

Sudden flaky alopecia, occasional scalp itching, a sensation of insects crawling on the scalp, a sensation of constant heat, irritability, anxiety, and restlessness. The tongue is red with scant coating, and the pulse is thready and rapid. Some cases will display hair loss of the eyebrows and beard in the later stages.

【Treatment Principle】

Cool blood and extinguish wind, nourish yin.

【Commonly Used Medicinals】

To cool blood and nourish yin, select *shēng dì huáng* (Radix Rehmanniae), *mǔ dān pí* (Cortex Moutan), *chì sháo* (Radix Paeoniae Rubra), *bái sháo* (Radix Paeoniae Alba), *sāng shèn* (Fructus Mori), *xuán shēn* (Radix Scrophulariae), and *tù sī zǐ* (Semen Cuscutae).

【Representative Formula】

Modified *Sì Wù Tāng* (四物汤) with *Èr Zhì Wán* (二至丸).

【Ingredients】

当归	dāng guī	15g	Radix Angelicae Sinensis
生地黄	shēng dì huáng	15g	Radix Rehmanniae
女贞子	nǚ zhēn zǐ	15g	Fructus Ligustri Lucidi
旱莲草	hàn lián cǎo	15g	Herba Ecliptae
牡丹皮	mǔ dān pí	15g	Cortex Moutan
赤芍	chì sháo	15g	Radix Paeoniae Rubra
山茱萸	shān zhū yú	12g	Fructus Corni
川芎	chuān xiōng	6g	Rhizoma Chuanxiong
菟丝子	tù sī zǐ	12g	Semen Cuscutae

Decoct in 500 ml of water until 100 ml of the decoction is left. Take warm, twice a day.

【Formula Analysis】

Shēng dì huáng (Radix Rehmanniae) is sweet and warm with a rich flavor and a moist nature. It enters the liver and kidney channels, nourishes yin and blood, tonifies the kidney and replenishes essence. It is also the first choice for nourishing blood and so serves as the chief medicinal in this formula. *Dāng guī* (Radix Angelicae Sinensis) is sweet, acrid and warm. Entering the liver, heart, and spleen channels; it also nourishes and invigorates blood, and so serves as the deputy medicinal. *Dān pí* (Cortex Moutan) and *chì sháo* (Radix Paeoniae Rubra) nourish blood and boost yin. *Chuān xiōng* (Rhizoma Chuanxiong) invigorates blood and moves qi. *Nǚ zhēn zǐ* (Fructus Ligustri Lucidi), *hàn lián cǎo* (Herba Ecliptae), *shān zhū yú* (Fructus Corni), and *tù sī zǐ* (Semen Cuscutae) act to supplement the kidney, replenish essence, and nourish the hair.

【Modifications】

➢ For insomnia, add *jué míng zǐ* (Semen Cassiae) 15g, and *cí shí* (Magnetitum) 30g to subdue yang and quiet the spirit.

➢ For sudden and severe hair loss due to prevalent wind-heat, add *Shéng Yìng Yǎng Zhēn Dān* (神应养真丹). Or add *tiān má* (Rhizoma Gastrodiae) 10g and *bái fù zǐ* (Rhizoma Typhonii) 10g to extinguish wind.

➢ For severe pruritus, add *bái xiān pí* (Cortex Dictamni) 12g, *suān zǎo rén* (Semen Ziziphi Spinosae) 12g, and *bǎi jiāng cán* (Bombyx Batryticatus) 8g to dispel wind, quiet the spirit, and relieve itching.

(4) Dual Deficiency of Qi and Blood

【Syndrome Characteristics】

This type of alopecia often occurs soon after childbirth or as a result of chronic illness. This type of alopecia has a gradual onset, range and severity. Signs and symptoms include a bright and soft-looking scalp, with scattered patches of alopecia, and hair falling out easily with a slight touch. Others include pale lips, palpitations, lethargy, weakness, shortness of breath, dizziness, blurred vision, and somnolence or insomnia. The tongue is light red with a thin white coating, and the pulse is thready and weak.

【Treatment Principle】

Fortify the spleen and benefit qi, nourish blood.

【Commonly Used Medicinals】

Dǎng shēn (Radix Codonopsis), *huáng qí* (Radix Astragali), *bái zhú* (Rhizoma Atractylodis Macrocephalae) and *fú líng* (Poria) fortify the spleen and benefit qi. *Zhì hé shǒu wū* (Radix Polygoni Multiflori Praeparata cum Succo Glycines Sotae), *huáng jīng* (Rhizoma Polygonati), *shú dì huáng* (Radix Rehmanniae Praeparata) and *bái sháo* (Radix Paeoniae Alba) nourish blood and yin.

【Representative Formula】

Modified *Rén Shēn Yǎng Róng Tāng* (人参养荣汤).

【Ingredients】

党参	dǎng shēn	15g	Radix Codonopsis
黄芪	huáng qí	15g	Radix Astragali
白术	bái zhú	12g	Rhizoma Atractylodis Macrocephalae
茯苓	fú líng	12g	Poria
制何首乌	zhì hé shǒu wū	15g	Radix Polygoni Multiflori Praeparata cum Succo Glycines Sotae
黄精	huáng jīng	15g	Rhizoma Polygonati
熟地黄	shú dì huáng	15g	Radix Rehmanniae Praeparata
当归	dāng guī	12g	Radix Angelicae Sinensis
白芍	bái sháo	12g	Radix Paeoniae Alba
甘草	gān cǎo	3g	Radix et Rhizoma Glycyrrhizae

Decoct in 500 ml of water until 100 ml of the decoction is left. Drink warm, twice a day.

【Formula Analysis】

As the chief herbs in the formula, *dǎng shēn* (Radix Codonopsis) and *huáng qí* (Radix Astragali) are used together to benefit qi and nourish blood. *Bái zhú* (Rhizoma Atractylodis Macrocephalae) and *fú líng* (Poria) fortify the spleen and leach out dampness. They also support *dǎng shēn* (Radix Codonopsis) in benefiting qi and nourishing the spleen. *Dāng guī* (Radix Angelicae Sinensis) and *bái sháo* (Radix Paeoniae Alba) nourish blood and harmonize the nutritive, and also assist *shú dì huáng* (Radix Rehmanniae Praeparata) to nourish the heart and liver. *Bái zhú* (Rhizoma Atractylodis Macrocephalae), *fú líng* (Poria), *dāng guī* (Radix Angelicae Sinensis) and *bái sháo* (Radix Paeoniae Alba) are the deputy herbs. *Huáng qí* (Radix Astragali) fortifies the spleen and benefits qi, while *zhì hé shǒu wū* (Radix Polygoni Multiflori Praeparata cum Succo Glycines Sotae) and *huáng jīng* (Rhizoma Polygonati) tonify the kidney and replenish essence to nourish the hair.

【Modifications】

➢ In cases of palpitation and insomnia, add *wǔ wèi zǐ* (Fructus Schisandrae Chinensis) 9g, *bǎi hé* (Bulbus Lilii) 12g, and *bǎi zǐ rén* (Semen Platycladi) 15g to nourish the heart and quiet the spirit.

➢ In cases of heat induced by blood deficiency, add *huáng qín* (Radix Scutellariae) 9g, *mǔ dān pí* (Cortex Moutan) 12g, *shú dì huáng* (Radix Rehmanniae Praeparata) 15g, and *shēng dì huáng* (Radix Rehmanniae) 15g to clear heat and cool the blood.

Additional Treatment Modalities

1. Chinese Patent Medicine

(1) *Bān Tū Wán* (斑秃丸)

4 grams, three times a day. It can tonify blood, dispel wind, and nourish yin and hair. Indicated for yin and blood deficiency with exuberant wind in the upper body.

(2) *Rén Shēn Yǎng Róng Wán* (人参养荣丸)

6 grams, twice a day. It can tonify qi, nourish blood, and quiet the spirit. Indicated for for deficiency of qi and blood.

(3) *Qī Bǎo Měi Rán Dān* (七宝美髯丹)

6 grams, three times a day. It nourishes blood and tonifies the kidney to darken hair color and promote hair regrowth. Indicated for for blood and kidney deficiency.

(4) *Shēng Fà Wán* (生发丸)

One pill, three times a day. It can tonify qi and blood and nourish the liver and kidney. Indicated for qi and blood deficiencies of the liver and kidney.

(5) *Shí Quán Dà Bǔ Gāo* (十全大补膏)

20-25 grams, three times a day. Indicated for qi and blood deficiency syndromes.

(6) *Dāng Guī Piàn* (当归片)

Three pills, three times a day. Indicated for deficiency of the liver and kidney.

(7) *Qǐ Jú Dì Huáng Wán* (杞菊地黄丸)

6 grams, two or three times a day. Indicated for deficiency of the liver and kidney.

2. Acupuncture and Moxibustion

(1) Acupuncture

【Point Selection】

DU 20	*bǎi huì*	百会
DU 23	*shàng xīng*	上星
DU 19	*hòu dǐng*	后顶
ST 36	*zú sān lǐ*	足三里
SP 6	*sān yīn jiāo*	三阴交

【Point Modification】

➢ Blood heat

GB 20	*fēng chí*	风池
SP 10	*xuè hǎi*	血海
ST 36	*zú sān lǐ*	足三里

➢ Blood stasis

LR 3	*tài chōng*	太冲
PC 6 to TE 5	*nèi guān to wài guān*	内关透外关

| SP 6 | sān yīn jiāo | 三阴交 |
| BL 17 | gé shù | 膈俞 |

> Blood Deficiency

BL 18	gān shù	肝俞
BL 23	shèn shù	肾俞
KI 3	tài xī	太溪
SP 10	xuè hǎi	血海
SP 6	sān yīn jiāo	三阴交

For severe itching, add GB 20 (*fēng chí*) and DU 14 (*dà zhuī*).

For insomnia, add *sì shéng cōng* (EX-HN 1) and *shén mén* (TF 4).

For alopecia of the temple region, add ST 8 (*tóu wéi*) and GB 8 (*shuài gǔ*).

For poor appetite, add CV 12 (*zhōng wǎn*) and ST 36 (*zú sān lǐ*).

For eyebrow alopecia, needle *yú yāo* (EX-HN 4) through to SJ 23 (*sī zhú kōng*).

For oily hair, add GV 23 (*shàng xīng*).

【Manipulation】

Treat excess syndromes with draining methods, and treat deficient syndromes with tonifying methods. Needles are retained for 30 minutes and manipulated 3-5 times. One treatment every two days; 10 treatments constitute one course of treatment.

(2) Surround Needles for Promoting Hair Regrowth

【Point Selection】

Alopecia area.

【Manipulation】

The scalp is sterilized with proper antiseptic procedures. Filiform needles are inserted obliquely into the subcutaneous region around the alopecia area at about a 15 degree angle. Needles are retained for 30 minutes and manipulated 3-5 times. One treatment every two days;

10 treatments constitute one course of treatment.

(3) Ear Acupuncture
【Point Selection】

lung	CO14	*fèi*	肺
kidney	CO10	*shèn*	肾
shen men	TF4	*shén mén*	神门
sympathetic	AH6a	*jiāo gǎn*	交感
endocrine	CO18	*nèi fēn mì*	内分泌
spleen	CO13	*pí*	脾

【Manipulation】

Needles are manipulated 5-6 times during the 30 minute treatment session. One treatment every two days; 10 treatments constitute one course of treatment.

(4) Plum-blossom Needle
【Point Selection】

ashi points			阿是穴（斑秃区）
GB 20		*fēng chí*	风池
LU 9		*tài yuān*	太渊
PC 6		*nèi guān*	内关
AH 9		*yāo dǐ zhuī*	腰骶椎
DU 2		*yāo shù*	腰俞

【Point Modification】

➢ For alopecia on both temple regions, add ST 8 (*tóu wéi*).

➢ For alopecia on the vertex, add DU 20 (*bǎi huì*), GV 21 (*qián dǐng*), and DU 19 (*hòu dǐng*). For severe itching, add GB 20 (*fēng chí*) and DU 16 (*fēng fǔ*).

➢ For kidney deficiency, add BL 23 (*shèn shù*) and KI 3 (*tài xī*).

【Manipulation】

Tap the affected area with a plum-blossom needle with moderate stimulation until the area is red or bleeding slightly. Electrical stimulation may be administered. (Injections at the points can be used initially, followed by treatment with an electric plum-blossom needle device.) Treat every day or every two days. Fourteen treatments constitute one course of treatment.

(5) Massage

【Point Selection】

BL18	gān shù	肝俞
BL 23	shèn shù	肾俞
SP 10	xuè hǎi	血海
SP 6	sān yīn jiāo	三阴交
GB 20	fēng chí	风池
DU 20	bǎi huì	百会
EX-HN 3	yìn táng	印堂

【Manipulation】

Massage the above acupuncture points. Apply ginger and massage into the affected areas. Treat once a day for 20 minutes. Scalp massages can promote blood circulation and tissue blood perfusion in order to invigorate blood, transform stasis, and generate new blood to promote hair growth.

(6) Scalp Self-massage

【Manipulation】

The patient is asked to sit with legs apart, parallel with the shoulders. They are then instructed to open their hands and comb the head with their fingers from the forehead towards the occipital region. They are also asked to massage the top of the head towards both temples and the occipital regions. Then they are to massage and press the scalp with all ten fingers. Finally, using the thumb and index finger they are instructed to massage acupuncture points *tài yáng* (EX-HN 5), GB 20 (*fēng chí*), and

DU 16 (*fēng fǔ*). The massage ends with some light tapping around the scalp.

(7) Exercises to Beautify the Hair
【Instructions】

Sit on the floor with legs 30 cm apart, grab the calves, and bend forward to the floor 12 times. Sitting cross-legged and facing the east, make a fist with the thumbs inside, and hold the breath. Next, cover the ears with the palms for a minute. Then, crossing the hands at the back of the head, grab the ears and pull. Finally, gently pull the hair on the temples. This exercise should be performed once or twice each day.

This exercise is from the *Treatise on the Pathogenesis and Manifestations of All Disease* (诸病源候论, *Zhū Bìng Yuán Hòu Lùn*). It promotes qi and blood circulation, and nourishes the essential qi to darken and brighten the hair. Ancient people believed that bending over to touch the ground could act to regulate the function and flexibility of the spinal column, which also helps to promote essential qi and blood circulation to nourish the hair. Also, pulling of the ears and hair also act to benefit qi and blood circulation.

3. External Applications

(1) Ginger or Garlic

Cut or grind garlic or *shēng jiāng* (Rhizoma Zingiberis Recens) into small pieces. Older pieces of *shēng jiāng* (Rhizoma Zingiberis Recens) and garlic with a single head with a purple top are ideal. The garlic or ginger should be rubbed on the affected areas to create a sensation of heat. Treat 3-4 times a day.

(2) Herbal Juice

Fresh *hàn lián cǎo* (Herba Ecliptae) is washed and squeezed to extract its juice. The juice is applied to the affected area. Treat 3-4 times a day.

(3) Mixing Herbs with Vinegar

The powder of *bàn xià* (Rhizoma Pinelliae) or *chuān wū* (raw Radix Aconiti) is mixed with vinegar and then applied to the affected area. Apply each morning and evening.

(4) Herbal Tincture

Soak *Shēng Fà Wū Fà Dīng* (生发乌发酊) in a 75% concentration of alcohol for 14 days. Then drain the liquid and apply to the affected areas.

西洋参	xī yáng shēn	20g	Radix Panacis Quinquefolii
三七	sān qī	5g	Radix et Rhizoma Notoginseng
红花	hóng huā	10g	Flos Carthami
川芎	chuān xiōng	20g	Rhizoma Chuanxiong
丹参	dān shēn	15g	Radix et Rhizoma Salviae Miltiorrhizae
甘草	gān cǎo	10g	Radix et Rhizoma Glycyrrhizae
花椒	huā jiāo	8g	Pericarpium Zanthoxyli

Apply 3-5 times every day.

(5) Herbal Washing Therapy

Decoct the following herbs twice, 20 minutes each time. Mix the 2 batches and rub it into the affected areas for 15-20 minutes, twice daily.

何首乌	hé shǒu wū	30g	Radix Polygoni Multiflori
夜交藤	yè jiāo téng	30g	Caulis Polygoni Multiflori
枸杞子	gǒu qǐ zǐ	20g	Fructus Lycii
黄柏	huáng bǎi	20g	Cortex Phellodendri Chinensis
旱莲草	hàn lián cǎo	20g	Herba Ecliptae
龙胆草	lóng dǎn cǎo	20g	Radix et Rhizoma Gentianae
白鲜皮	bái xiān pí	15g	Cortex Dictamni
苦参	kǔ shēn	30g	Radix Sophorae Flavescentis
干姜	gān jiāng	20g	Rhizoma Zingiberis

| 地肤子 | *dì fū zǐ* | 20g | Fructus Kochiae |
| 辣椒干 | *là jiāo gān* | 100g | dried red pepper |

4. Simple Prescriptions and Empirical Formulas

(1) *Dōng chóng xià cǎo* (Cordyceps) Wine (冬虫夏草酒)

Soak *dōng chóng xià cǎo* (Cordyceps) 30g in 200 ml of white wine for a week. Apply to the affected area daily.

(2) 30% *Bǔ Gǔ Zhī* (Fructus Psoraleae) Tincture (30%补骨脂酊)

Soak *bǔ gǔ zhī* (Fructus Psoraleae) 30g in 100 ml of 75% alcohol. The alcohol tincture is applied to the affected area 2 times a day.

(3) 25% *Huā Jiāo* (Pericarpium Zanthoxyli) Tincture (25%花椒酊)

Soak *huā jiāo* (Pericarpium Zanthoxyli) 25g in 100 ml of 75% alcohol. The alcohol is applied to the affected areas 3 times a day.

(4) 10% *Jīn Sù Lán* (henry chloranthus) Tincture (金粟兰酊)

Soak *jīn sù lán* (henry chloranthus) 10g in 100 ml of 75% alcohol. The alcohol is applied to the affected areas daily.

(5) Soak fresh *cè bǎi yè* (Cacumen Platycladi) 90g and *shān nài* (Rhizoma Kaempferiae) 45g in 700 ml of 75% alcohol for 7 to 10 days. *Shēng jiāng* (Rhizoma Zingiberis Recens) is then cut into pieces, dipped into the alcohol, and applied to the alopecia area. Apply 2 times a day.

(6) Cut and soak *bān máo* (Mylabris) 7g, *gǔ suì bǔ* (Rhizoma Drynariae) 12g, *bǔ gǔ zhī* (Fructus Psoraleae) 12g, and fresh *cè bǎi yè* (Cacumen Platycladi) 30g in 500 ml of 75% alcohol or white wine for 1 week. The liquid is applied to the local area until the local skin turns reddish.

(7) Soak *shé chuáng zǐ* (Fructus Cnidii) 500g, *bǎi bù* (Radix Stemonae 250g), *huáng bǎi* (Cortex Phellodendri Chinensis) and *míng fán* (Alumen) 20g in 340-440 ml of 75% alcohol for 1-10 weeks. Drain the liquid and add

20 ml of glycerol for every 100 ml of liquid. The mixture is applied to all affected areas.

(8) Decoct *sāng bái pí* (Cortex Mori) 100g into 300 ml of water for 30 minutes. Use the decocted liquid to wash the hair. Use twice daily.

(9) Decoct *shēng dì huáng* (Radix Rehmanniae) 30g, *hé shǒu wū* (Radix Polygoni Multiflori) 30g, *hēi zhī ma* (Semen Sesami Nigrum) 50g and *liǔ shù zhī* (willow) 50g. Wash the hair with this decoction three times a day, and then cover with a dry towel for 30 minutes to allow the decoction to seep into the hair and scalp.

(10) Decoct *tòu gǔ cǎo* (Caulis Impatientis) 45g and use the decocted liquid to wash the hair for 20 minutes each time. Use everyday. Do not wash the herbal decoction out of the hair.

PROGNOSIS

Alopecia can be effectively treated if an accurate diagnosis is followed by the correct treatment and proper management during the early stages. However, middle-aged patients have more difficult regaining full recovery than younger patients. It is more difficult to recover large patches of alopecia areata in the elderly. Minor patches of alopecia in the occipital regions can spontaneously recover, but should be monitored for recurrence. Alopecia areata in the temporal regions above the ears is also more difficult to treat. Alopecia areata due to a genetic predisposition usually develops into a chronic condition with a poor prognosis. Serpentine alopecia, which is rarely seen in the clinic, usually occurs among children and only sometimes with adults. It usually affects the occipital region, temporal region and hairline. These patients typically have unusual constitutions and not responsive to most interventions and therapies. Most of these cases lead to alopecia totalis even before adolescence, and show very low recovery rates. In fact, complete recovery is rarely seen in the clinic. When combined with nevus flammeus, prognosis is even worse.

The disease course for alopecia areata varies from a few months to a few years. Generally speaking, the course tends to be longer for hair loss on larger regions, long term conditions, and for alopecia due to multiple factors. Alopecia areata generally tends to spontaneously recover, but then recur. Even after hair has regrown following clinical treatment, about 33%-50% of these patients will have recurrence, typically within a year. Nearly 30% of the cases lead to alopecia universalis, especially in adolescents. Alopecia areata may develop into alopecia universalis within several weeks, but typically it takes about two years. The cases that do not turn into alopecia universalis within 5 years seem to have less difficulty recovering when treated in clinic.

PREVENTIVE HEALTHCARE

Alopecia areata belongs under the category of dermatopathy (dermatological diseases). This condition damages the aesthetic appearance and therefore also associated with psychological and mental factors. Improving the daily lifestyle will increase the benefits of clinical treatment and other therapies.

Regulation of Emotional and Mental Health

Patients are advised to alternate work with rest, maintain a level of contentment, and to avoid stress, pessimism, sorrow, and anger. They are encouraged to be optimistic and confident during the course of treatment. The practitioner should not alter the formula frequently, but instead remain consistent with the selected applications.

Lifestyle Modification

Patients should keep their hair clean, and avoid using strong alkaline-based soaps or shampoos, also avoiding hair products containing strong chemicals. It is not recommended to dry the hair with a blow dryer, or to dye the hair.

Dietary Recommendation

Patients should maintain a diverse diet, eliminate bad eating habits, and avoid consuming only their favorite foods. Alopecia areata is closely related to the diet, and the recommended foods are based on pattern differentiation of the skin condition.

Generally speaking, alopecia areata is closely related to emotional tension. In additional to regulating the emotions, foods that can calm the spirit should be added into the diet such as *bǎi hé* (Bulbus Lilii), *lián zǐ* (Semen Nelumbinis), *mǔ lì* (Concha Ostreae) and *suān zǎo rén* (Semen Ziziphi Spinosae). Patients who are deficient in blood and essence should eat foods high in protein to tonify the blood and essence such as sea cucumber, prawn, sleeve-fish, black sesame, and walnut seed. For phlegm and stasis stagnation patterns, luffa cylindrical (loofah), herring, lotus root, brown sugar, and shepherd's purse are recommended to unblock the collaterals and transform phlegm.

The following herbs and foods benefit the hair and can be used for dietary therapy: *hēi zhī ma* (Semen Sesami Nigrum), *sāng shèn* (Fructus Mori), *hé shǒu wū* (Radix Polygoni Multiflori), *nǚ zhēn zǐ* (Fructus Ligustri Lucidi), *gǒu qǐ zǐ* (Fructus Lycii), *shān yào* (Rhizoma Dioscoreae), *dà zǎo* (Fructus Jujubae), *hēi dòu* (Semen Sojae Nigrum), *táo rén* (Semen Persicae), *jú huā* (Flos Chrysanthemi), lean meat, mutton, carrot, spinach, liver, cabbage, fish, chicken, lotus root, asparagus, lettuce, *shān zhā* (Fructus Crataegi), eggplant, kelp, and *hēi zǎo* (Diospyros lotus).

(1) *Cè Bǎi Sāng Shèn* Ointment (侧柏桑椹膏)

Ingredients: *Cè bǎi yè* (Cacumen Platycladi) 50g, *sāng shèn* (Fructus

Mori) 200g, and honey 50g.

Cè bǎi yè (Cacumen Platycladi) is steamed for 20 minutes. Discard the dregs and add *sāng shèn* (Fructus Mori). Then decoct over low heat for half an hour. Discard the dregs, drain the liquid and add honey to make an ointment.

This ointment is used for alopecia areata due to the stirring of wind due to blood heat with symptoms of sudden and rapid flaky alopecia, shiny hair, visible hair follicles, irritability, restlessness, thirst, constipation, insomnia, excessive dreaming. The tongue is red with a red tip and a thin yellow coating. The pulse is thready, or thin and rapid.

(2) *Jú Huā Hàn Lián Yǐn* (菊花旱莲饮)

Decoct *jú huā* (Flos Chrysanthemi) 10g and *mò hàn lián* (Herba Ecliptae) 5g. Drink frequently in place of tea. Suitable for alopecia areata due to the stirring of wind due to blood heat.

(3) Stewed Soft-shelled Turtle

Ingredients: Soft-shelled turtle (about 500g), *nǚ zhēn zǐ* (Fructus Ligustri Lucidi) 10g, *gǒu qǐ zǐ* (Fructus Lycii) 10g, and 10 pieces of *dà zǎo* (Fructus Jujubae). Wash the turtle, cut it into pieces and place them in water for boiling. Then decoct *nǚ zhēn zǐ* (Fructus Ligustri Lucidi), *gǒu qǐ zǐ* (Fructus Lycii), and *dà zǎo* (Fructus Jujubae) for 20 minutes until 20 ml of liquid remains. Discard the dregs and drain. Then pour 20 ml of the decocted liquid with other condiments into the pot with the turtle, and stew until cooked.

This recipe treats alopecia areata due to blood and essence deficiency with symptoms of dry and brittle hair, hair that grows but easily falls out, pale complexion, vertigo, tinnitus, dizziness, insomnia, excessive dreaming, aching lumbus and limp limbs, a pale tongue with scant coating, and a thready weak pulse.

(4) *Sāng Shèn Shēng Fà Gāo* (桑椹生发膏)

Ingredients: *Sāng shèn* (Fructus Mori) 200g, *hé shǒu wū* (Radix Polygoni Multiflori) 150g, *shú dì huáng* (Radix Rehmanniae Praeparata) 300g and an optional amount of honey. The ingredients may be are decocted three times in water. Add honey to a concentrated decoction to make an ointment. This preparation is suitable for blood and essence deficiency.

(5) *Gǒu Qǐ (Fructus Lycii)* Fried with Sea Cucumber

Ingredients: Sea cucumber 300g, *gǒu qǐ* (Fructus Lycii) 15g and *sāng shèn* (Fructus Mori) 10g. Cut the sea cucumber into long narrow pieces, fry them with hot oil and condiments, and simmer them over a low flame until the boiling. Then add steamed *gǒu qǐ* (Fructus Lycii) and *sāng shèn* (Fructus Mori). At the end, add starch juice to the decoction. Suitable for blood and essence deficiency.

(6) *Hóng Yóu Gē ǒu Piàn* (红油鸽藕片)

Ingredients: Fresh lotus root 500g, *hóng huā* (Flos Carthami) 5g and dove meat 200g. *Hóng huā* (Flos Carthami) is first fried in sesame oil. Discard the dregs and drain the oil. Wash the fresh lotus root and cut into pieces, then fry with dove meat. Finally, pour the *hóng huā* (Flos Carthami) oil onto the dove meat. This medicinal recipe is appropriate for long term alopecia areata, alopecia totalis, or alopecia universalis due to blood stasis manifesting with a stabbing painful scalp, head distention, headache, and a dark or dusky complexion.

(7) *Táo Rén (Semen Persicae) Zhī Ma* Gruel (桃仁芝麻粥)

Ingredients: White rice 200g, *táo rén* (Semen Persicae) 10g, *zhī ma* (Semen Sesami Nigrum) 10g, and *hēi dà dòu* (Semen Sojae Nigrum) 10g are cooked into a gruel or porridge.

Indicated for alopecia areata associated with blood stasis.

(8) *Hóng Táng Shān Zhā* Liquid (红糖山楂饮)

Ingredients: *Shān zhā* (Fructus Crataegi) 200g and brown sugar 20g. Decoct *shān zhā* (Fructus Crataegi) and add a little sugar. Indicated for alopecia areata with patterns of blood stasis.

(9) *Hóng Zǎo Qǐ Zǐ* and Egg Soup (红枣杞子煲鸡蛋)

Decoct *hóng zǎo* (Fructus Jujubae) 10 pieces, *gǒu qǐ zǐ* (Fructus Lycii) 30g, and two eggs. Remove the eggshell and simmer the egg for several minutes. Consume both the eggs and soup. This medicinal recipe is suitable for post-partum blood deficiency types of alopecia.

(10) *Pú Gōng Yīng* with *Wū Dòu* (蒲公英煲乌豆)

Decoct together *pú gōng yīng* (Herba Taraxaci) 60g, and *wū dòu* (Semen Sojae Nigrum) 1000g. Discard the *pú gōng yīng* (Herba Taraxaci) and add crystal sugar. Take several times daily. This medicinal recipe treats various types of alopecia with signs and symptoms of internal heat.

CLINICAL EXPERIENCE OF RENOWNED PHYSICIANS

Empirical Formulas

1. *Gù Shèn Shēng Fà Tāng* (固肾生发汤) (Liang Jian-hui)

【Ingredients】

熟地黄	shú dì huáng	30g	Radix Rehmanniae Praeparata
何首乌	hé shǒu wū	15g	Radix Polygoni Multiflori
木瓜	mù guā	20g	Fructus Chaenomelis
党参	dǎng shēn	15g	Radix Codonopsis
丹参	dān shēn	20g	Radix et Rhizoma Salviae Miltiorrhizae
枸杞子	gǒu qǐ zǐ	15g	Fructus Lycii
桑椹子	sāng shèn	20g	Fructus Mori
川芎	chuān xiōng	5g	Rhizoma Chuanxiong
黑芝麻	hēi zhī ma	30g	Semen Sesami Nigrum
女贞子	nǚ zhēn zǐ	15g	Fructus Ligustri Lucidi

【Indications】

Alopecia areata, alopecia totalis or alopecia universalis due to insufficiency of the liver and kidney with qi and blood deficiency.

【Modifications】

➢ For senile patients, add *yín yáng huò* (Herba Epimedii), *jīn yīng zǐ* (Fructus Rosae Laevigatae), and *bā jǐ tiān* (Radix Morindae Officinalis).

➢ For female patients, add *lù jiǎo jiāo* (Colla Cornus Cervi), *ē jiāo* (Colla Corii Asini), and *mò hàn lián* (Herba Ecliptae).

➢ For children, add *shān yào* (Rhizoma Dioscoreae), *lóng yǎn ròu* (Arillus Longan), and *fú líng* (Poria).

(Zhu Ren-kang, et al. Syndrome Differentiation and Treatment of Alopecia Areata (脱发证治). *Journal of Traditional Chinese Medicine* (中医杂志)1986, (12):11)

2. Bǔ Shèn Yǎng Xuè Tāng (补肾养血汤) (Liu Hui-min)

【Ingredients】

桑寄生	sāng jì shēng	24g	Herba Taxilli
女贞子	nǚ zhēn zǐ	15g	Fructus Ligustri Lucidi
枸杞子	gǒu qǐ zǐ	15g	Fructus Lycii
菟丝子	tù sī zǐ	12g	Semen Cuscutae
酸枣仁（生、炒各半）	suān zǎo rén	30g (15g dry-fried)	Semen Ziziphi Spinosae
地肤子	dì fū zǐ	12g	Fructus Kochiae
当归	dāng guī	9g	Radix Angelicae Sinensis
橘络	jú luò	9g	Vascular Aurantii
刺蒺藜	cì jí lí	9g	Fructus Tribuli
白鲜皮	bái xiān pí	9g	Cortex Dictamni
土茯苓	tǔ fú líng	9g	Rhizoma Smilacis Glabrae
天麻	tiān má	9g	Rhizoma Gastrodiae
茜草根	qiàn cǎo gēn	9g	Radix et Rhizoma Rubiae
五味子	wǔ wèi zǐ	6g	Fructus Schisandrae Chinensis
防风	fáng fēng	6g	Radix Saposhnikoviae

Recipe for external use:

【Ingredients】

鲜芝麻花	xiān zhī má huā	90g	nettleleaf meehania (fresh)
鲜鸡冠花	xiān jī guān huā	60g	Flos Celosiae Cristatae (fresh)

Cut the flowers into pieces and soak them in white wine for 2 weeks. Shake the bottle frequently throughout the 2 weeks. Filter the liquid and soak with 1.5g camphor. Apply to the affected area 2-3 times every day.

【Indications】

Deficiency of liver and kidney, and wind dryness due to blood deficiency.

【Modifications】

➢ For insomnia, add *suān zǎo rén* (dry-fried Semen Ziziphi Spinosae) and *wǔ wèi zǐ* (Fructus Schisandrae Chinensis) to nourish the heart and quiet the spirit.

➢ For spleen-stomach disharmony, add *jú luò* (Vascular Aurantii), *tǔ fú líng* (Rhizoma Smilacis Glabrae), and *bái zhú* (Rhizoma Atractylodis Macrocephalae) to regulate the spleen and stomach.

(Dai Qi. *Medical Cases of Liu Hui-min* (戴岐·刘惠民医案) Jinan: Shandong Science and Technology Press.1979.369)

3. Shén Yìng Yǎng Zhēn Tāng (神应养真汤) (Cheng Zhen)

【Ingredients】

熟地黄	shú dì huáng	15g	Radix Rehmanniae Praeparata
菟丝子	tù sī zǐ	15g	Semen Cuscutae
桑椹	sāng shèn	15g	Fructus Mori
旱莲草	hàn lián cǎo	20g	Herba Ecliptae
何首乌	shǒu wū	15g	Radix Polygoni Multiflori
当归	dāng guī	15g	Radix Angelicae Sinensis
黄芪	huáng qí	30g	Radix Astragali
白芍	bái sháo	15g	Radix Paeoniae Alba

女贞子	nǚ zhēn zǐ	15g	Fructus Ligustri Lucidi
川芎	chuān xiōng	10g	Rhizoma Chuanxiong

【Indications】

Malnourishment of the hair due to liver and kidney deficiency with qi and blood deficiency.

【Modifications】

➤ For palpitations and insomnia, add *suān zǎo rén* (Semen Ziziphi Spinosae) 15g, and *yuǎn zhì* (Radix Polygalae) 15g.

(Zhang Jun Ting. Editor-in-chief. *Classics of Chinese Medicine Diagnostic Skill* (中医诊疗特技精典). Beijing: Chinese Ancient Medical Books Publishing House,1994.620)

4. *Gǒu Qí Huáng Qí Tāng* (枸杞黄芪汤) (Luo Yu-guo)

【Ingredients】

枸杞子	gǒu qǐ zǐ	20g	Fructus Lycii
生黄芪	huáng qí	60g	Radix Astragali
熟地黄	shú dì huáng	15g	Radix Rehmanniae Praeparata
菟丝子	tù sī zǐ	20g	Semen Cuscutae
柏子仁	bǎi zǐ rén	20g	Semen Platycladi
当归	dāng guī	15g	Radix Angelicae Sinensis
党参	dǎng shēn	30g	Radix Codonopsis
升麻	shēng má	10g	Rhizoma Cimicifugae
柴胡	chái hú	10g	Radix Bupleuri
炙远志	yuǎn zhì	10g	Radix Polygalae (fried with liquid)
北五味子	wǔ wèi zǐ	15g	Fructus Schisandrae Chinensis
制何首乌	zhì hé shǒu wū	30g	Radix Polygoni Multiflori Praeparata cum Succo Glycines Sotae

【Indications】

Alopecia caused by deficiency of the liver and kidney with exhaustion of yin and blood.

(Zhu Ren-kang. Syndrome and Treatment of Alopecia (脱发证治).

Journal of Traditional Chinese Medicine (中医杂志).1986, (12):11)

5. Shēng Fà Wán (生发丸) (Shi Guan-qing)

【Ingredients】

蒸何首乌	hé shǒu wū	30g	Radix Polygoni Multiflori (prepared)
当归	dāng guī	15g	Radix Angelicae Sinensis
桃仁	táo rén	10g	Semen Persicae
红花	hóng huā	9g	Flos Carthami
赤芍	chì sháo	10g	Radix Paeoniae Rubra
柏子仁	bǎi zǐ rén	12g	Semen Platycladi
生地黄	shēng dì huáng	15g	Radix Rehmanniae
旱莲草	hàn lián cǎo	30g	Herba Ecliptae
怀牛膝	niú xī	12g	Radix Achyranthis Bidentatae
夏枯草	xià kū cǎo	15g	Spica Prunellae
甘草	gān cǎo	6g	Radix et Rhizoma Glycyrrhizae

【Indications】

Scattered flaky alopecia or alopecia totalis due to essence and blood deficiency, liver and kidney deficiency and blood stasis.

(Lu Xiang-zhi. Editor-in-chief. *Famous Formulas of Renowned TCM Doctors* (中国名医名方). Beijing: China Medical Science and Technology Press, 1991.110)

Selected Case Studies

1. Case Studies of Zhang Zhi-li: Liver, Kidney and Blood Deficiency

Ms. Shu, female, age 43.

【Initial Visiton】

September 5th, 1991.

The patient came into the clinic and reported that 5 months ago, she began to feel itching and pain on her scalp soon after dyeing the color of her hair. The hair began to fall out in patches. She tried Chinese medicine and biomedicines, as well as *Shēng Fà Jīng* (生发精) for external use, but they had little effect. The hair on her eyebrows and body began to fall out as well. She also reported thirst, poor appetite, insomnia, and excessive dreaming, as well as delayed scant menstruation.

Physical examination showed that three-fourths of her hair had fallen out, with sparse eyebrow hairs and a shiny scalp with sparse and brittle hair. Her hair would fall out with the slightest touch. The tongue was pale with a thin white tongue coating, and the pulse was deep and thready.

【Pattern Differentiation】

Alopecia due to deficiency of the liver, kidney and blood.

【Treatment Principle】

Tonify the liver and kidney, nourish blood.

【Prescription】

当归	dāng guī	10g	Radix Angelicae Sinensis
白芍	bái sháo	10g	Radix Paeoniae Alba
川芎	chuān xiōng	10g	Rhizoma Chuanxiong
夜交藤	yè jiāo téng	30g	Caulis Polygoni Multiflori
熟地黄	shú dì huáng	10g	Radix Rehmanniae Praeparata
女贞子	nǚ zhēn zǐ	30g	Fructus Ligustri Lucidi
菟丝子	tù sī zǐ	15g	Semen Cuscutae
黑桑椹	sāng shèn	15g	Fructus Mori
黑芝麻	hēi zhī ma	15g	Semen Sesami Nigrum
天麻	tiān má	10g	Rhizoma Gastrodiae
白术	bái zhú	10g	Rhizoma Atractylodis Macrocephalae
茯苓	fú líng	10g	Poria
石菖蒲	shí chāng pú	30g	Rhizoma Acori Tatarinowii
钩藤	gōu téng	10g	Ramulus Uncariae Cum Uncis
丹参	dān shēn	15g	Radix et Rhizoma Salviae Miltiorrhizae
鸡血藤	jī xuè téng	30g	Caulis Spatholobi

External use: *Shēng Fà Jiàn Fà Dīng* (生发健发酊).

【Second Visit】

After taking the prescription for one month, her hair stopped falling out and sleep also improved. Light colored brown hair began to regrow slightly on the temporal region. There was no obvious improvement in the eyebrow region. Also, the patient reported fullness and oppression in the chest and abdomen after eating.

The former prescription was modified by removing *jī xuè téng* (Caulis Spatholobi) and *gōu téng* (Ramulus Uncariae Cum Uncis), and adding *chén pí* (Pericarpium Citri Reticulatae) 10g, *zhǐ qiào* (Fructus Aurantii) 10g, and *bái zhǐ* (Radix Angelicae Dahuricae) 10g.

After taking the above prescription for two months, her appetite improved and most of the hair regrew. Her eyebrows had grown back, and her menstruation was regular.

(An Jia-feng. Editor-in-chief. *Selected Dermatopathy Cases from Zhang Zhi-li* (张志礼皮肤病医案选). Beijing: The People's Medical Publishing House, 1994.229)

2. Case Studies of Dong Jian-hua: Liver and Kidney Yin Deficiency

Mr. Huang, male, age 42.

【Initial Visit】

April 4th, 1983.

The patient's hair began to turn white and fall out in patches more than one year previously. After receiving therapy, the hair regenerated. However, it started to fall out again in April 1982. Other signs included a depressed mood, a red tongue with a yellow coating, and a deep, thready and wiry pulse.

【Pattern Differentiation】

Liver and kidney yin deficiency, and depressed internal fire.

【Treatment Principle】

Nourish yin, clear heat, and purge fire.

【Prescription】

生地黄	shēng dì huáng	10g	Radix Rehmanniae
熟地黄	shú dì huáng	10g	Radix Rehmanniae Praeparata
黑芝麻	hēi zhī ma	10g	Semen Sesami Nigrum
牡丹皮	mǔ dān pí	10g	Cortex Moutan
山栀子	shān zhī zǐ	10g	Fructus Gardeniae
侧柏叶	cè bǎi yè	10g	Cacumen Plateycladi
冬青子	dōng qīng zǐ	10g	Ilicis Chinensis Semen
白芍	bái sháo	10g	Radix Paeoniae Alba
旱莲草	hàn lián cǎo	10g	Herba Ecliptae
地骨皮	dì gǔ pí	10g	Cortex Lycii
生牡蛎（先煎）	shēng mǔ lì	20g	Concha Ostreae (decoct first)
制何首乌	zhì hé shǒu wū	15g	Radix Polygoni Multiflori Praeparata cum Succo Glycines Sotae

【Second Visit】

After ten doses, the rate of hair loss decreased. The tongue was red with a thin yellow coating, and the pulse was thready and wiry.

The former prescription was modified as follows:

黑芝麻	hēi zhī ma	10g	Semen Sesami Nigrum
冬青子	dōng qīng zǐ	10g	Ilicis Chinensis Semen
旱莲草	hàn lián cǎo	10g	Herba Ecliptae
地骨皮	dì gǔ pí	10g	Cortex Lycii
山药	shān yào	10g	Rhizoma Dioscoreae
熟地黄	shú dì huáng	10g	Radix Rehmanniae Praeparata
玄参	xuán shēn	10g	Radix Scrophulariae
侧柏叶	cè bǎi yè	10g	Cacumen Plateycladi
当归	dāng guī	10g	Radix Angelicae Sinensis
制何首乌	zhì hé shǒu wū	15g	Radix Polygoni Multiflori Praeparata cum Succo Glycines Sotae
黄精	huáng jīng	20g	Rhizoma Polygonati
牡丹皮	mǔ dān pí	6g	Cortex Moutan

After 30 doses, new hair began to grow, all the hair appearing black. The alopecia had almost completely resolved.

(Dong Jian-hua. Four Empirical Cases of Alopecia Areata (斑秃验案四则). *New Journal of Traditional Chinese Medicine* (新中医),1985, (11): 28-29)

3. Case Studies of Xuan Guo-wei : Qi and Yin Deficiency

Ms. Chai, female, age 37.

【Initial Visit】

December 3rd, 1996.

The patient's scalp, eyebrow, armpit and pubic hair had fallen out. Two years previously, her hair began to fall out rapidly, without obvious reason. Although she took prednisone and thyroid tablets, her hair loss could not be controlled. Hair loss also spread to the eyebrows, armpit, and pubic region. Accompanying symptoms included vexation, dry mouth, poor appetite, poor sleep, and profuse dreaming. Her urination and bowel movements were normal. Examination showed a red shiny scalp, sparse hairs in the eyebrow, armpit and pubic areas. the tongue was pale red with a thin and white coating. The pulse was wiry, thready and weak.

【Pattern Differentiation】

Qi and yin depletion causing malnourishment of the hair.

【Treatment Principle】

Benefit qi and nourish yin.

【Prescription】

太子参	tài zǐ shēn	15g	Radix Pseudostellariae
玄参	xuán shēn	15g	Radix Scrophulariae
生地黄	shēng dì huáng	20g	Radix Rehmanniae
女贞子	nǚ zhēn zǐ	20g	Fructus Ligustri Lucidi
桑椹	sāng shèn	20g	Fructus Mori
桑叶	sāng yè	10g	Folium Mori
酸枣仁	suān zǎo rén	15g	Semen Ziziphi Spinosae
生黄芪	shēng huáng qí	15g	Radix Astragali
白芍	bái sháo	30g	Radix Paeoniae Alba

煅牡蛎（先煎）	duàn mǔ lì	30g	Concha Ostreae (prepared) (decoct first)
天麻	tiān má	12g	Rhizoma Gastrodiae
川芎	chuān xiōng	6g	Rhizoma Chuanxiong
甘草	gān cǎo	6g	Radix et Rhizoma Glycyrrhizae

External use: *Wū Fà Shēng Fà Dīng* (乌发生发酊).

【Second Visit】

After taking the above prescription for one month, a large amount of vellus hair (short, fine hair; also known as "peach fuzz") had grown on the scalp. Hair loss on the eyebrows, as well as in the armpit and pubic regions stopped, and slight hair growth was observed. Her complaints of vexation, dry mouth, poor sleep, and profuse dreaming had improved. The former prescription was modified by removing *xuán shēn* (Radix Scrophulariae) 20g, and adding *shú dì huáng* (Radix Rehmanniae Praeparata) 20g.

After two more months, the vellus hair on the scalp had become thicker and blacker. The hair on her eyebrows, as well as of the armpit and pubic regions grew back almost completely. The patient was instructed to take *Yì Fà #3 Oral Liquid* (益发三号口服液) with *Wū Fà Shēng Fà Dīng* for external use to complete the treatment.

(Chen Da-can, Fan Rui-qiang and Lu Chuan-jian. Editors-in-chief. *Essentials of Clinical Chinese Medicine in Dermatopathy* (皮肤病中医临证精粹). Guangzhou: Guangdong Science and Technology Press, 2001:182)

Discussions

1. Deng Tie-tao on Pattern Differentiation and Treatment

Professor Deng Tie-tao believes that liver and kidney deficiency patterns are the basis for all types of alopecia. The liver stores blood, and the kidney stores essence. Since the kidney is mother of the liver, essence and blood generate each other. When the liver and kidney are well-nourished, there will be sufficient essence and blood to nourish the hair, and hair will grow vigorously. On the contrary, if the liver cannot store blood and the kidney-essence is damaged, hair will lose nutrition and fall out. Therefore, Dr. Deng often selects *dì huáng* (Radix Rehmanniae), *huáng jīng* (Rhizoma Polygonati) and *sāng shèn* (Fructus Mori) to nourish the kidney and essence, as well as *hēi dòu* (Semen Sojae Nigrum), *dāng guī* (Radix Angelicae Sinensis), *hé shǒu wū* (Radix Polygoni Multiflori), and *sāng shèn* (Fructus Mori) to nourish the liver and generate blood. In particular, he regards *hēi dòu* (Semen Sojae Nigrum), *hé shǒu wū* (Radix Polygoni Multiflori), *dì huáng* (Radix Rehmanniae) and *sāng shèn* (Fructus Mori) as essential medicinals in the treatment of alopecia areata. Dr. Deng prefers to add medicinals that invigorate the blood to the above tonifying medicinals, such as *jī xuè téng* (Caulis Spatholobi). Together, they tonify essence and blood while also moving and generating blood. In all, they are nourishing but not cloying.

Dr. Deng also believes that qi deficiency plays an important role in the pathogenesis of alopecia areata. Qi is the commander of the blood, and blood is the mother of qi. Blood deficiency leads to qi deficiency, and qi deficiency can cause blood deficiency as well. If lung qi is insufficient, its function of diffusion is compromised, and therefore the lung cannot support the skin and hair, which could further aggravate the alopecia and makes hair regrowth more difficult. Moreover, lung qi deficiency is the reason that patients with blood deficiency could also appear with symptoms of qi deficiency. Therefore, the treatment strategy should enrich the blood and tonify qi together. Nourishing blood can provide the substance and foundation for hair growth, while tonifying qi provides the energy and force for the body to grow hair. Enriching the blood complements tonifying the body's qi, and this treatment principle obtains the best results. *Huáng qí* (Radix Astragali), *wǔ zhuǎ lóng* (Radix Ipomoeae Cairicae), *tài zǐ shēn* (Radix Pseudostellariae) and *fú líng* (Poria) are used for nourishing the lung and spleen in order to tonify qi.

Deng also aims to strengthen the liver and kidney deficiency which often leads to yin deficiency and internal heat. Manifestations include insomnia with profuse dreaming, restlessness, a thready and rapid pulse, and a red tongue with red prickles at the tip. For liver and kidney deficiency with internal heat, *Èr Zhì Wán* (二至丸) is recommended to nourish yin and clear internal heat. To avoid yin deficiency generating internal heat, Deng suggests tonifying medicinals that are not too warm, hot or dry. He prefers to select mildly warm medicinals instead. Therefore, *tài zǐ shēn* (Radix Pseudostellariae) and *wǔ zhuǎ lóng* (Radix Ipomoeae Cairicae) have become his favorite medicinals to tonify qi; and he sometimes replaces *shú dì huáng* (Radix Rehmanniae Praeparata) with *shēng dì huáng* (Radix Rehmanniae).

Acupuncture and topical alcohol applications can also enhance local blood circulation and improve qi and blood circulation by stimulating the local affected areas. Methods include:

(1) Apply brandy to the head and feet each morning, especially on the affected areas.

(2) For large areas of alopecia, prick to bleed the affected areas.

(Deng Zhong-yan. Doctor Deng Tie-tao's Experience in the Treatment of Alopecia Areata (邓铁涛教授治疗斑秃的经验). *New Journal of Traditional Chinese Medicine* (新中医), 1981, (2):16-17)

2. Dong Jian-hua on Kidney and Blood Tonification

As the *Inner Canon of the Yellow Emperor* (黄帝内经 , *Huáng Dì Nèi Jīng*) states: "The kidney stores essence, governs the bones, and engenders marrow". "If kidney qi is excess, hair grows and teeth change; if kidney qi is deficiency, hair loss and teeth are dry and dead." There is also a theory that essence and blood promote each other. If essence and blood are exuberant, hair is also abundant. Dong believes that the hair's source of vitality stems from the kidney, while the hair's source of nutrition is from the blood. Therefore, treatment for alopecia areata should emphasize tonifying the kidney and blood with formulas such as modified Èr Zhì Wán (二至丸).

Collected Exegesis of Medical Formulas (医方集解 , *Yī Fāng Jí Jiě*) states: "Èr Zhì Wán (二至丸), is a formula of *shaoyin* herbs. *Nǚ zhēn zǐ* (Fructus Ligustri Lucidi) is sweet and neutral, which nourishes liver and kidney. *Hàn lián cǎo* (Herba Ecliptae) is sweet and cold, and also enters the kidney channel to enrich essence. Together, they not only tonify the lower [*zang*] and but also nourish the upper [body]. In all, the formula made of the two herbs can nourish yin and darken the hair color." Dr. Dong explains that *Èr Zhì Wán* (二至丸) is nourishing but not slimy; it tonifies the body without causing dryness; it cools the blood and moistens dryness. Undoubtedly, it is an effective formula for alopecia areata. When it is used with *hé shǒu wū* (Radix Polygoni Multiflori), *huáng jīng* (Rhizoma Polygonati), *dāng guī* (Radix Angelicae Sinensis), *shú dì huáng* (Radix Rehmanniae Praeparata), *shēng dì huáng* (Radix Rehmanniae), *gǒu qǐ zǐ* (Fructus Lycii) and *hēi zhī ma* (Semen Sesami Nigrum) to enhance its nourishing effects, and *mǔ dān pí* (Cortex Moutan), *cè bǎi yè* (Cacumen Platycladi) and *zhī zǐ* (Fructus Gardeniae) to purge heat, cool the blood and moisten the dryness, better clinical results could be achieved.

In *Golden Mirror of the Medical Tradition* (*Yī Zōng Jīn Jiàn,* 医宗金鉴), it is recommended to use wind-dispelling medicinals like *qiāng huó* (Rhizoma et Radix Notopterygii) to treat alopecia areata. However, according to Dong's long term clinical practice and experience, he points out that the theory is not practical in clinic. He explains that wind-dispelling medicinals such as *qiāng huó* (Rhizoma et Radix Notopterygii) are always acrid and warm. Therefore, it can easily consume and stir the blood, which would further aggravate the deficiency of essence and blood in alopecia areata patients. So Dong suggests TCM doctors should not choose wind-dispelling medicinals like *qiāng huó* (Rhizoma et Radix Notopterygii) to treat alopecia areata.

(Dong Jian-hua. Four Experiences of Alopecia Areata (斑秃验案四则). *New Journal of Traditional Chinese Medicine* (新中医), 1985, (11): 28-29)

3. Lü Zhi-lian on Alopecia Areata with Deficiency Predominating

The early stages of alopecia areata develop slowly and gradually with hair loss ranging from the size of a small coin to a large coin. Accompanying symptoms include insomnia, tinnitus, and poor memory. They are always categorized as deficiency syndromes. For patients with strong constitutions manifesting as sudden abrupt hair loss in large regions in round or irregular shapes or even total hair loss, they are categorized as excess syndromes. There is typically more deficiency than excess. However, purely deficient patients are seldom seen in the clinic (except in cases of alopecia post-chemotherapy or post-radiation therapy). Furthermore, deficiency syndromes often co-exist with excess syndromes. Doctor Lü often chooses Wang Qing-ren's *Tōng Qiào Huó Xuè Tāng* (通窍活血汤) with modifications to treat the disease.

【Prescription】

当归	dāng guī	12g	Radix Angelicae Sinensis
赤芍	chì sháo	10g	Radix Paeoniae Rubra
川芎	chuān xiōng	6g	Rhizoma Chuanxiong
桃仁	táo rén	10g	Semen Persicae
葱根	cōng gēn	5枚	Allii Fistulosi Radix
鲜姜	xiān jiāng	5片	Rhizoma Zingiberis Recens
红枣	hóng zǎo	15g	Fructus Jujubae
香白芷（代麝香）	xiāng bái zhǐ	12g	Radix Angelicae Dahuricae(instead of shè xiāng)
红花	hóng huā	3g	Flos Carthami

熟地黄	*shú dì huáng*	15g	Radix Rehmanniae Praeparata
生地黄	*shēng dì huáng*	15g	Radix Rehmanniae

【Modifications】

➤ For deficiency syndromes, add *hàn lián cǎo* (Herba Ecliptae) 15g, *gǒu qǐ zǐ* (Fructus Lycii) 12g, *hēi zhī ma* (Semen Sesami Nigrum) 15g, *shān zhū yú* (Fructus Corni) 12g, *zhì hé shǒu wū* (Radix Polygoni Multiflori Praeparata cum Succo Glycines Sotae) 20g.

➤ For excess syndromes, add *dān shēn* (Radix et Rhizoma Salviae Miltiorrhizae) 15g, *dài zhě shí* (Haematitum) 15g, *cì jí lí* (Fructus Tribuli) 15g, and *yì yǐ rén* (Semen Coicis) 30g.

To promote mental health, advise the patient to maintain a steady mood. Also, daily dietary nutrition should be maintained or improved.

(Cheng Jue-tang. Editor-in-chief. *Contemporary Chinese Medicine Experts Gathering Experience 1* [中国当代中医专家临床经验荟萃（一）]. Beijing: Academy Press (学苑出版社), 1997.410)

4. Li Shu-tang on Draining Water, Dispelling Dampness, and Transforming Phlegm

Alopecia areata in the clinic is most often differentiated as exuberant wind with blood dryness, and blood stasis obstructing the collaterals. However, Dr. Li finds that these patterns do not apply to most pediatric patients. In fact, he finds that they have metabolic fluid disorders, which lead to phlegm and thin mucus retention in the hair follicles. Therefore, the treatment principles of promoting water flow, dispelling dampness, and transforming phlegm are most appropriate for alopecia areata.

Soak *yuán huā* (Flos Genkwa) 5g and *gān suì* (Radix Kansui) 5g in 50g of rice vinegar for 24 hours, and then add 50g of water; soaking for another 24 hours. Dip a cotton ball into the liquid and apply 3-4 times to the affected area everyday. Pain will stop, and hair will grow after the medicine is applied regularly. For some patients, it achieves good effects after one week of treatment. This liniment is appropriate for children or adults who have alopecia areata due to phlegm and thin mucus.

(Wang Feng-qi. Editor-in-chief. *Integrated Techniques of Famous Chinese Doctors* (中华名医特技集成). Beijing: China Medical Science and Technology Press, 1993.221)

PERSPECTIVES OF INTEGRATIVE MEDICINE

Challenges and Solutions

Diagnosing alopecia areata is not difficult, but focus should be placed on the correct treatment. Alopecia areata can be easy to cure if biomedicines are combined with Chinese medicine, with internal and external therapies also combined. The difficulties are how to prevent simple alopecia areata from worsening and developing into more serious conditions such as alopecia totalis, and how to cure critical alopecia, pediatric alopecia and recurrent alopecia.

CHALLENGE #1: HOW TO PREVENT PROGRESSION

Alopecia areata is divided into 3 stages: the active stage, the resting stage, and the ambiguous stage. Managing alopecia areata during the active stage is central to proper treatment. First, it is important to determine the condition is in the active stage. Moreover, treatment should focus on preventing simple alopecia areata from developing into critical alopecia. Although the pathogenesis is not completely clear, dysfunctions within the immune system are considered to be the primary cause. It is also related to psychological factors, vasomotor activity, genetics, endocrine disorders, infections, and environmental toxins. Immune and endocrine functions of the hypophysis, thyroid, and adrenal glands can also be tested to help determine cause and treatment.

Secondly, more complicated cases combine psychotherapy, topical applications, and oral medications. Cases of alopecia areata induced by psychological factors should receive psychological support or psychotherapy. Particularly during the active stage, patients should alleviate all mental stressors, develop confidence in the medical interventions, cooperate with the doctor, and comply with treatment protocols.

Topical drug treatments can penetrate hair follicles and the surrounding skin. It will be absorbed into the bloodstream and circulate to the hair follicles everywhere in the body, which is beneficial for even treating simple alopecia areata. For patients with simple alopecia areata, it is crucial to use internal herbal medicine during the active stage, even if it seems like an uncomplicated condition. Although local treatment can be effective and rapid, it is also important to prevent the side effects of atrophoderma (shrinking of the scalp skin). When there are no results using standard treatment, topical applications that inhibit hormones should be applied.

CHALLENGE #2: HOW TO TREAT CRITICAL ALOPECIA

Critical alopecia is a type of alopecia areata that affects one-third of the scalp, or has lasted at least one year. It progresses quickly, permeating larger regions. Preferred herbs for treatment would activate blood circulation, eliminate blood stasis, dispel wind and open the channels. Based on the syndrome, high doses of herbs can be used to invigorate qi such as *huáng qí* (Radix Astragali) and *gāo lì shēn* (Radix Ginseng Coreensis). Meanwhile, regulating the lung is effective for patients who have had lengthy yet unsuccessful treatments. Cortical hormones used early on can be controlled, but attention should be paid to its contraindications. The practitioner should weigh the advantages and disadvantages of glucocorticosteroid treatments, and offer patients appropriate supportive drugs or therapies. Before treating patients with hormones, practitioners must consider the possibility of higher relapse rates, longer courses of treatment, the inability to discontinue or reduce dosage amounts, treatments that can last 2 or more years (without any results), and a lack of response due to tolerance. Research shows that cortical hormones sustained at low dosages are effective in treating most critical alopecia types in the early stages. The keys for success in using cortical hormones are thorough patient clinical examinations, assessment of its appropriate use, and the considerations of contraindication. Furthermore, early application of mucosal protective agents is recommended to protect the gastrointestinal mucosa. Meanwhile, morning administration of corticosteroids are recommended for some conditions to reduce side effects and promote efficacy of the drug. Immunomodulators such as thymiosin, levamisole, and isoprinosine can also be chosen. Total efficacy improves when internal therapy is utilized with the support of external therapies.

CHALLENGE #3: HOW TO TREAT PEDIATRIC ALOPECIA

Pediatric alopecia has its own unique characteristics. First, it is unusual to find psychological causes except for childhood panic attack. Second, there are frequent recurrences, which easily develop into alopecia totalis. Weak congenital constitutions generally involve spleen and kidney deficiencies as the main causes. Therefore, the main treatment principle is to strengthen the spleen and nourish the kidney. Also focus on regulating the spleen and stomach to promote its function of transformation and production. It is important also to pay attention to potential bacterial and fungicidal infections, and to treat it with herbal lotions as necessary. Infections can destroy a patient's hair follicles, making them vulnerable to recurrences. Anti-inflammatory medicines are also effective in treating pediatric alopecia. Cortical hormones certainly benefit pediatric alopecia, but only external uses are applied in order to minimize side effects. Immunomodulators are also used as supplemental intervention, if necessary.

CHALLENGE #4: HOW TO REDUCE RECURRENCE

The main cause for recurrence is related to drug dependence, lingering inflammation around the hair follicle, and sudden termination or severe dosage reduction. The efficacy of alopecia treatment is in direct proportion to the length of treatment. Treatments lasting 3-6 months are the most successful. To stabilize the effect of treatment after hair has grown back, it is important to completely eliminate inflammation around the hair follicle to control the disease. Even after clinical success, the medicine should be not discontinued abruptly, but rather the dosage should be slowly tapered over a period of time. The patient should continue to take medicines to regulate the immune function, which would also reduce the likelihood of recurrence.

Insight from Empirical Wisdom

There is a wealth of information on the Chinese medicine treatment of alopecia areata, especially with the use of these 3 following topical applications:

(1) The use of *máo jiāng* [*gǔ suì bǔ*] (Rhizoma Drynariae) and capsicum frutescens tincture for eternal application.

(2) Baking fresh *shēng jiāng* (Rhizoma Zingiberis Recens) and applying it to the area.

(3) The use of plum blossom needles for tapping on affected areas.

These methods are examples of ordinary and simple ways of applying Chinese medicine techniques. Combined therapies are recommended, such as the combining of internal and external medicines, of psychotherapy and medication, and of biomedicines with Chinese medicine. Internal treatments are based on the concept of whole-body regulation, depending on the presenting syndrome. External treatments act directly on the affected areas, and can provide temporary relief of symptoms. These two methods supplement each other, treating both symptom and root.

Psychotherapy also plays a crucial role, especially if the alopecia was caused by psychological factors. During the active stages, ask the patient to alleviate stress, trust in the medical interventions, and remain compliant to the treatment. Chinese medicinals regulate the whole body and can take a slow gradual effect. However, its effect lasts for a longer period of time with few side effects. Western medicine has an immediate, significant and direct impact on medical conditions, but it can also display toxic side effects. Results tend to be temporary, and recurrence is high. Combining biomedicines with Chinese medicine seems to be a logical approach to use the strengths of both while offsetting the weakness of each system. This approach could increase the overall effect while also decreasing side effects. This is found to be more favorable than using western medicine or Chinese medicine alone.

Recently, experts in China and in other countries have found that combining therapies is the best solution for alopecia areata. More research indicates that combining herbs with other therapeutic modalities create a synergistic effect on alopecia areata. This data implies further evidence that combined therapies are better than single therapies. Internal herbal therapy should not be overlooked for simple alopecia areata, flaky alopecia areata, and especially for critical alopecia, alopecia totalis, and alopecia universalis during the active stages. These latter conditions need more intensive treatments. Although there are pathogenic and various factors that can complicate the conditions, the pathology lies not just locally on the skin, but rather in a systemic dysfunction of the entire body. The concept of holism is clinically important when the goal is to balance the yin and yang of the body in order to regulate immunological functions. Multiple therapies, interventions, and comprehensive treatments should all be utilized to increase efficacy. Essentially, the focus should be on creating treatments based on syndrome differentiation, combining internal and external treatments, and the joining of biomedicine with Chinese medicine. Most patients will typically recover with standard treatment, but customizing and combining various therapies can bring beneficial results, especially for difficult and unusual cases. The most concrete methods include the following:

1. Percussopunctation and TDP Equipment

After proper sterilization, tap selected affected areas, GV 20 (*bǎi huì*), and GB 2 (*fēng chí*) with a plum blossom needle. Tap lightly on red and swollen areas, and tap with medium strength on areas with no improvement to make that area slightly red with increased blood flow to the local tissues. Heavy tapping should be applied to depressed areas of the scalp for 3-5 minutes to induce slight bleeding. This treatment is followed by placing a preheated TDP lamp on the affected areas. Keep the TDP lamp at a distance of 20-30 cm or within a comfortable distance. Treat 15-20 minutes each time, twice a week.

2. External Application of *Yì Fà B* Tincture and Hormones

Grind 150mg prednisone into powder, and mix with 100ml of *Yì Fà B* Tincture (益发 B 外用酊) [pharmaceutical preparations dispensed in Guangdong Provincial Hospital of Traditional Chinese Medicine]. Shake, and dip a fresh piece of ginger into the mixture and apply to the affected areas. Tap and rub the medication into the scalp until it turns red. Use this tincture three times a day.

It is relatively difficult to treat vital alopecia. Biomedicine finds that corticosteroid certainly resolves the disease, but its clinical application is controversial since alopecia areata has unpleasant aesthetic effects. Long term and systemic application of the hormone can have significant side effects. Some have used hormones like prednisolone, triamcinolone, or acetonide for local and symptomatic treatments using topical applications. However, the efficacy significantly decreases if corticosteroids are applied on more than 50% of the scalp during an active stage. In some cases, hair will not grow, or side effects of scalp atrophy will occur. Thus, the use of hormones in treating alopecia areata has always been of clinical concern.

Yì Fà B Tincture is one of the medications made in the Guangdong Provincial Hospital of Traditional Chinese Medicine, and it contains *rén shēn yè* (Folium Ginseng), *huā jiāo* (Pericarpium Zanthoxyli), *huáng qí* (Radix Astragali), and *hóng huā* (Flos Carthami). Research has indicated that this tincture dilates capillaries in the superficial dermis layers of rabbits, increases blood circulation, improves local microcirculation, increases nutrition reaching the hair follicles and also promotes hair growth and regeneration. The results using the tincture in the clinic are quite successful. *Yì Fà B* Tincture and hormones are used together or with other comprehensive therapies to treat vital alopecia, with good results and no side effects of scalp atrophy.

In addition to the above combination of therapies, Chinese medicine syndrome differentiation is strongly emphasized.

First, herbs that are warm and dry should be applied most carefully. Hair is the manifestation of blood, which belongs to yin. Regardless of whether the diagnosis is spleen deficiency or liver deficiency, it is important to apply nourishing and moistening herbs. Alopecia areata is mainly caused by internal wind, not pathogenic exterior wind. Therefore, herbs that expel exterior wind are contraindicated to avoid injuring yin fluids.

Second, it is necessary to differentiate deficiency syndromes from excess syndromes. Generally speaking, excess often occurs in adolescent patients with strong constitutions. Most of the time, the excess syndromes of alopecia areata manifest with a sudden onset, shiny hair, red and lustrous complexion, normal tongue, and a wiry tight excess pulse. Postpartum patients usually have deficiency syndromes and also those recovering from serious or long-term illnesses. In prolonged illnesses, patients show patches of hair loss, pale complexion, low energy, soreness and weakness of the lower back, fatigue, withered and yellowish-colored hair, and a pale tongue with a soggy, thin or weak pulse.

Thirdly, blood deficiency, blood stasis, and blood heat syndromes should be clearly differentiated. A patient with blood deficiency has a yellowish complexion, fatigue, weakness, withered and yellowish-colored hair, pale lips and tongue, and a thin weak pulse. A patient with blood heat has a shiny red complexion, sudden alopecia, an itchy scalp as if insects were crawling and biting, shiny and oily scalp, emotional depression, irritability, a red tongue, and a wiry rapid pulse. A patient with blood stasis has a red, lustrous or darker complexion, dark lips, headaches, a purple tongue with dark sides, or a dark tongue with petechiae and ecchymosis, and a wiry or rough pulse.

Previous generations of doctors have advanced our understanding by introducing concepts of excessive wind and blood deficiency in the diagnosis alopecia areata. Other treatment principles of alopecia areata include nourishing blood, dispelling wind, invigorating the spleen and reinforcing the kidney. Abundant clinical data has been gathered in recent years to illustrate those other syndromes that can affect alopecia. Blood deficiency, blood heat, blood stasis and kidney deficiency can induce alopecia, and thus should be treated accordingly by nourishing blood and qi, cooling blood and calming interior wind, activating blood and regulating qi, tonifying the kidney, and replenishing essence. Factors of age, weakness, post-illness deficiencies, postpartum hemorrhaging, overthinking, and fatigue, poor diet, and emotional depression can certainly lead to liver, kidney, essence and blood deficiency. Herbal prescriptions should be based on the correct diagnosis and syndrome. The primary principles to treat the symptom and root of alopecia areata are mainly tonifying deficiencies; such as benefiting the kidney to supplement essence, and also nourishing and regulating the blood.

If alopecia totalis or alopecia universalis patients cannot regrow hair even after the above treatments methods, other means should be taken:

Every evening, redden the scalp with one of 2 methods:

(1) Tap the alopecia areas with a plum blossom needle.

(2) Place a warm compress (using a moist towel) on the scalp. Then place a layer of cotton over the towel and carefully pour *Wū Fà Shēng Fà Dīng* (乌发生发酊) onto the layer of cotton. Be sure that the liquid does not drip. Then secure it with a bath cap throughout the night until the next morning. With burning or other obvious discomfort, remove the herbal solution. Try again after the burning or discomfort subsides. This method is most effective for patients whom have had no hair growth for a long period of time.

(3) Grind 24 egg shells into powder. Mix the following herbs with the powder to make a cream: *táo rén* (Semen Persicae) 20g, *xìng rén* (Semen Armeniacae Amarum) 15g, *zào jiǎo* (Spina Gleditsiae) 15g, *dà huáng* (Radix et Rhizoma Rhei) 7.5g, *liú huáng* (Sulfur) 7.5g and lard (raw) 150g. Apply the cream on the affected areas. Recommend the patient wear a white hat for seven days. Thin and white vellus hairs should grow after 7 days of application. Two weeks later, apply the cream again. If there is burning or itching with the application of the cream, remove the cream immediately to avoid damage to the skin.

Summary

Alopecia areata is a very common dermatological disease. Fast paced living, increased work stress, and environmental pollution all influence the immune system, ultimately affecting the superficial skin areas, especially in alopecia areata patients. Due to higher standards of living, more patients actively seek out treatment for this condition.

1. Syndrome Differentiation and Pathogenesis

The general pathogenesis of alopecia areata involves patterns of wind created by blood heat, qi and blood deficiency, liver depression and blood stasis, or liver and kidney deficiency. Research in recent years shows that there exist an increased number of etiologies and syndromes. There are three predominating syndromes: kidney deficiency, blood deficiency, and blood stasis. These three patterns can be addressed easily in clinic, and are also conducive to further research. However, alopecia is also closely related with blood stasis. Fatigue can create heart and spleen deficiency which can generate disruption of the seven emotions, depression, qi and blood stagnation, ultimately leading to blood stasis. Hair loss can also be due to poor nutrition. Biomedical theory purports that psychological stress and poor immune functioning can result in an insufficiency of nutrients reaching the hair follicles. The interrelationship between alopecia, psychological states, and body fluids should be further researched.

Liver and kidney deficiency is still the most commonly seen syndrome in the clinic. The primary premise that the liver stores blood, the blood nourishes the hair, and that the kidney stores essence. This supports the common diagnosis of liver and kidney deficiency, and also the lack of nutrients reaching the hair. The primary treatment principle includes tonifying the kidney to supplement essence, nourishing blood, and regulating blood. The most frequently used Chinese herbs in formulas for the internal treatment of alopecia areata are: *dāng guī* (Radix Angelicae Sinensis), *hé shǒu wū* (Radix Polygoni Multiflori), *shú dì* (Radix

Rehmanniae Praeparata), *chuān xiōng* (Rhizoma Chuanxiong), *gǒu qǐ zǐ* (Fructus Lycii), *huáng qí* (Radix Astragali), *tù sī zǐ* (Semen Cuscutae) and *nǚ zhēn zǐ* (Fructus Ligustri Lucidi). All of these herbs reinforce the kidney, replenish essence, nourish blood, and stimulate hair growth.

The analysis on 25 hair-darkening formulas and 82 herbs in the *Prescriptions of Universal Benefit* (*Pǔ Jì Fāng*, 普济方) showed that hair loss at the scalp and beard can best be treated with kidney tonic herbs. The most commonly used herbs in those formulas were: *shú dì huáng* (Radix Rehmanniae Praeparata), *shēng dì* (Radix Rehmanniae), *gǒu qǐ zǐ* (Fructus Lycii), *tù sī zǐ* (Semen Cuscutae), *huái niú xī* (Radix Achyranthis Bidentatae), *bǔ gǔ zhī* (Fructus Psoraleae), *fú líng* (Poria), *huáng jīng* (Rhizoma Polygonati) and *shān zhū yú* (Fructus Corni). Factors include age, weakness, deficiency after illnesses, postpartum hemorrhaging, overthinking, poor diet, and emotional depression. All of these factors contribute to liver, kidney, essence, and blood deficiencies. This is the premise for selecting herbal prescriptions.

2. Alopecia and Comprehensive Therapies

There is ample clinical data using internal herbal medicine and also external therapies such as *máo jiāng* [*gǔ suì bǔ*] (Rhizoma Drynariae), capsicum frutescens tincture, baked fresh *shēng jiāng* (Rhizoma Zingiberis Recens) for topical application, plum blossom needle techniques, and acupuncture. Traditional massage, *tuina*, and *qigong* can also be combined with herbal therapy as well. Analysis medical journal articles shows a strong emphasis on using both holistic concepts and all-inclusive therapies (such as acupuncture combined with topical treatments) when treating alopecia areata. The clinical recovery rate is always around 70%, while the overall effective rate is over 90%. Treatment principles mentioned in these journals often include: tonifying the kidney, nourishing and activating blood in order to nourish the hair follicle, improving hair growth by enhancing microcirculation, adjusting endocrine functions, and increasing immunological function.

Internal herbal therapy should not be overlooked for simple alopecia areata, flaky alopecia areata, and especially for critical alopecia, alopecia totalis, and alopecia universalis during the active stages. These latter conditions need more intensive treatments. Although there are various pathogenic factors that can complicate these conditions, the pathology lies not just locally at the hair follicle, but rather in a systemic dysfunction of the entire body. The concept of holism is clinically important when the goal is to balance yin and yang in order to regulate immunological functions. Multiple therapies, and interventions, and comprehensive treatments are advised to improve overall effects.

Combining of therapies is often used in chronic illnesses with unknown causes, or for conditions in which there are no available treatments. The purpose is to utilize multiple methods on the same patient in order to obtain the best results. Comprehensive therapies in alopecia areata treatment combine both internal and external medicine, psychotherapy and medication, and biomedicine with Chinese medicine. Internal treatment in Chinese medicine first requires clear syndrome differentiation in order to holistically regulate the body. External treatments act directly on the local affected areas to provide temporary relief of symptoms. Internal and external treatments supplement each other to treat both the symptom and root. Psychotherapy is particularly important when alopecia areata precipitated by psychological factors.

Many doctors have realized the importance of psychological factors in alopecia areata treatment. Psychological distress can lead to autonomic dysfunction, increased activity in the sympathetic nervous system, constriction of the capillaries, and compromised endocrine and immune systems, all which can hinder the delivery of sufficient nutrients to the hair follicle. Combining psychological support with medical treatments can ease a restless mind, stabilize emotional states, and relieve burdens. When necessary, psychological therapy may also increase the patient's confidence that the hair can regrow, and thereby improve the treatment outcomes. Current research confirms that the combination of herbs with other therapeutic modalities often create a synergistic effect.

The most effective therapies for alopecia areata should be investigated and clearly documented. Also, modern bioscience should be combined with new technologies. For example, corticosteroid medications with topical applications can be an effective method. New methods can be found in the ancient books of Chinese medicine, such as the Chinese medicated diet for hair growth and darkening of hair color. All alopecia areata patients have psychological distress to some degree. Thus, psychological support or rehabilitation can be necessary or even pivotal to recovery. Researching the methods of the ancient doctors would broaden and deepen the strength of medicine in treating alopecia areata. Delving into ancient records can also advance treatments and obtain greater success.

In recent years, comprehensive therapies have been widely adopted in the clinic, but it has not been gaining much attention from the general public. However, numerous medical reports show that various therapies are given to patients, but the compatibility between the different therapies or herbs are not observed. Without taking notice of the interactions between different interventions, therapies that synergistically blend together for greater therapeutic effect will be more difficult to identify. The treatments and understanding of herbal prescription for treating alopecia areata should follow these guidelines:

➢ Select herbs and therapies with different functions to enhance the overall effect by approaching the problem from different angles.

➢ Combine treatments to address both local and root problems.

➢ Avoid using herbs or therapies that have overlapping effects.

➤ Choose herbs or therapies that can be incorporated into a comprehensive treatment.

➤ Utilizing the least amount of therapies is important to maintain patient compliance.

3. Research on Various Alopecia Types

This sparse amount of data makes it difficult to understand its diagnosis and treatment. For example, critical alopecia areata can develop from simple alopecia areata into alopecia totalis or alopecia universalis. Investigating vital alopecia areata would also be helpful for diagnosis and treatment. It would provide information on how to control the active stages and decrease the likelihood of simple alopecia areata transforming into alopecia totalis or alopecia universalis. Conducting research offers a deeper understanding for the internal mechanism of recurrence and immunology. It can also provide a theoretical basis for comprehensive therapy, new treatment methods, broadened clinical perspectives, improved recovery rates, and shortened duration. Therefore, further research should focus on a breakthrough for critical alopecia areata, alopecia totalis, alopecia universalis, and recurrent alopecia areata.

Alopecia areata tends to heal spontaneously, especially during the recovery stage. Most scientific research designs do not distinguish cases in the active stage, resting stage or ambiguous stage. This ambiguity makes it difficult to assess the exact efficacy of each therapy. Past research seems to lack design that utilizes comparative and replicable research. Future research studies should have stricter design standards particularly for outcome measurements. Furthermore, there should be a focus on comparing the efficacy of biomedicine and Chinese medicine. It is important to select effective comprehensive therapies with optimal results that increase recovery rates for refractory alopecia.

4. Combining Corticosteroids with Chinese Medicinals

Corticosteroids are effective in treating critical alopecia areata, alopecia totalis and alopecia universalis. Zhang Jing-zheng gave 30-40 mg of prednisone for patients to take in the morning everyday for 40 days. Patients whose hair completely recovered gradually decreased their dosages within 4-6 months with eventual termination of the drug. Of the 36 cases treated, 19 cases were cured, 11 cases had improved outcomes, 4 were effective, and 15 relapsed. The overall effective rate was 94.4% and the recurrence rate was 44.1%.

Methylprednisolone pulse therapy was given to 45 cases outside of China with the following procedure: intravenous administration of 250 mg methylprednisolone, twice daily for three days as one course of treatment. If it was not effective or relapse occurred within 3-13 months after the first course, the patients were given one more course. Two days before and one week after the therapy, they took oral ranitidine 300 mg per day to prevent gastrointestinal side effects. Blood pressure, heart rate, and blood sugar were monitored during treatment. The results indicated that methylprednisolone pulse therapy was more effective for critical alopecia areata that was rapid, progressive, and related to multiple factors.

Others compared and researched the usages of corticosteroids. A small dosage of prednisone was used in the first (therapeutic) group. They took 10-20 mg in the morning every day for six weeks. The second group added local treatment (2% lidocaine 1 ml and prednisolone 1 ml) on the scalp in addition to the oral prednisone once a week with 1-2 applications each time. In the control group, the patients were treated with intermediate dosages of prednisolone, 30-40 mg everyday, three times a day. The patients were treated for six weeks. For patients with effective results, their dosages were gradually reduced until the corticosteroid was completely discontinued with a 4-6 months period. The results indicated that both therapies had significant results on alopecia areata. There was no difference in therapeutic time, recurrence time and recurrence rate between these two groups, but the side effects in therapeutic group was much smaller than in the control group. Once effective results were attained, the dosage was gradually reduced.

Based on the data mentioned above, the combination of biomedicine and Chinese medicine is more effective in treating critical alopecia areata, alopecia totalis, and alopecia universalis. However, it warrants further research on the appropriate dosage for effective outcomes and the reduction of side effects. The etiology of alopecia areata is still not clear. In biomedicine, this condition is related with decreased immune function, psychological factors, heredity, endocrine disorders, and local infections. However there are a few scholars that deny the involvement of the autoimmune system in alopecia areata, because it has not been proven conclusively. Moreover, autoimmune disorders have only been associated with a few patients. However, in some cases, the autoimmune system is involved, where patients were resistant to immune therapy treatment. Systematic use of corticosteroids cannot prevent alopecia areata from spreading or relapsing. Even after the hair has completely grown back, it will fall out again after the treatment ends. Long term and systemic application of this hormone cannot prevent its side effects. Therefore, cortical hormones should be used early on to control the condition, but one needs to pay attention its contraindications. The practitioner should weigh the advantages and disadvantages when prescribing cortical hormone treatment and offer other supportive therapies. Further studies should be conducted comparing different dosages of corticosteroid treatment and in combination with other therapy modalities. Comprehensive therapy should be used to enhance clinical effect as way to reduce the corticosteroid dosage and its side effects.

5. Descriptive Reports and Clinical Research

This kind of research can be limiting as Chinese medicine fails to utilize advanced methods of measurement in biomedicine. It is difficult to find specific guidelines and information for treatment, the process of hair growth, and medicines with high efficacy for hair growth. The affected areas of alopecia area are concentrated areas with abnormal immune mechanism. An infiltration of lymphocyte T cells in the follicle and surrounding areas has been confirmed.

Inflammatory factors and antigen cells play an important role in inflammation also. Research is needed to further interpret the pharmacological mechanism of Chinese external medicinals, including the effects of Chinese external medicinals on the immunoinflammatory reactions of the affected area. Other facts that require further investigation are the transdermal rates, distribution in the skin, and the metabolism and absorption rate of using pharmacodynamics and pharmacokinetics methods. Oral administration of Chinese patent drugs such as *Bān Tū* Pills (斑秃片), *Gù Shèn Shēng Fà* Pills (固肾生发片) and *Yǎng Xuě Shēng Fà* Capsules (养血生发胶囊) have shown significant effects. Traditional Chinese medicine preparations and single Chinese herb extracts such as pachymaran, ganoderma lucidum polysaccharide and lentinan are plant-based immunomodulators which effectively treat alopecia areata. However, the research on the immunopharmacology of Chinese herbs requires a deeper understanding. It is now necessary to research alopecia areata in both clinical settings and animal lab experimental settings to investigate the following processes: the effects of regulating the liver on alopecia areata's neuropeptide P, the impact of immunological function and cytokines when reinforcing liver and kidney, the relationship between the Chinese method of activating blood circulation and dissipating blood stasis on the obstruction of blood supply around the hair follicles, vascular endothelial growth factor, endothelial cell apoptosis, the pharmacodynamics of formulas and single herbs, and new Chinese herbal preparations such as the *Shēng Fà Dīng* (生发酊) spray. The research mentioned above will further open and expand laboratory studies and provide a new approach of Chinese medicine for alopecia areata. It would also provide the theoretical principles and scientific foundations for developing new drugs. This kind of research will lead to a thorough study of Chinese medicine.

SELECTED QUOTES FROM CLASSICAL TEXTS

Complete Compendium of Royal Surgeons—Category of Hair (疡医大全·头发门, *Yáng Yī Dà Quán: Tóu Fà Mén,*)

"生姜切片，探落发光皮上，数日即长。" "花椒四两，用白酒酿七日，早晚润秃处，其处自生"

"Cut *shēng jiāng* (Rhizoma Zingiberis Recens) into pieces, apply to the affected area of the shiny scalp. The hair will grow in a few days." "Four *liang huā jiāo* (Pericarpium Zanthoxyli) is brewed with alcohol for seven days. Apply the alcohol on the alopecia area every day and night, and the hair will grow."

Discussion of the Origins of the Symptoms of Disease—Symptoms of Ghost-Licked Head (诸病源候论·鬼舐头候, *Zhū Bìng Yuán Hòu Lùn: Guǐ Tiǎn Tóu Hòu*)

"人有风邪在于头，有偏虚处，则发秃落，肌肉枯死。或如钱大，或如指大，发不生，亦不痒，故谓之鬼舐头"。

"If pathogenic wind attacks deficient areas of the head, hair will fall out and the muscles will atrophy. The affected areas may be as big as copper cash or a finger, no hair grows and there is no itching. That is why it is called ghost-licked head."

Orthodox Manual of External Diseases—Glossy Scalp Wind (外科正宗·油风, *Wài Kē Zhèng Zōng: Yóu Fēng*)

"油风，乃血虚不能随气荣养肌肤，故毛发根枯，脱落成片，皮肤光亮，痒如虫行，此皆风热乘虚攻注而然，治当神应养真丹服之，外以海艾汤熏洗并效。"

"Glossy scalp wind is caused by blood deficiency which cannot nourish the skin with qi. Hence the hair root is withered, and the hair is flaky. The skin will be shiny and feel itchy as if insects were crawling on the skin. This is all induced by wind-heat taking the advantage of the weak areas. It should be treated with *Shén Yìng Yǎng Zhēn Dān* (神应养真丹) for internal use and *Hǎi Ài Tāng* (海艾汤) for steaming and washing."

Medical Bank Stone (医碥, *Yī Biǎn*)

"人身毫毛皆微而发独盛者，何也？百脉会于百会，血气上行而为之生发也。血气上行，必有所止，止而因复下行，则发为之卫。"

"Why is the body hair thinning while hair on the head is in exuberance? All meridians collect in *bǎi huì* (GV 20). Blood and qi rise to promote hair growth. When blood and qi rise, they will stop and then go downward, which is defensive qi."

Wondrous Lantern for Peering into the Origin and Development of Miscellaneous Diseases (杂病源流犀烛, *Zá Bìng Yuán Liú Xī Zhú*)

"毛发也者，所以为一身之仪表，而可险盛衰于冲任二脉者也。"

"Hair appears on the whole body, but its exuberance and debilitation are closely related to the penetrating and conception vessels."

Golden Mirror of the Medical Tradition—Key and Mastery of Surgery (医宗金鉴·外科心法要诀, *Yī Zōng Jīn Jiàn: Wài Kē Xīn Fǎ Yào Jué*)

"油风，此证毛发干焦，成片脱落，皮红光亮，痒如虫行，俗名鬼剃头。由毛孔开张，邪风乘虚袭入，以致风盛燥血，不能荣养毛发。宜服神应养真丹，以治其本；外以海艾汤洗之，以治其标。若能延年久，宜针砭其光亮之处，出紫血，毛发庶可复生。"

"Hair is dry and flaky in glossy scalp wind. The scalp is red, shiny and itchy like insects crawling on it, so its popular name is ghost shaving head. Hair follicles are open, and pathogenic wind invades to take advantage of the weak areas, which fail to nourish hair and induce exuberant wind and dry blood. We should use *Shén Yìng Yǎng Zhēn Dān* (神应养真丹) to treat its root, and wash it with *Hǎi Ài Tāng* (海艾汤) to treat the branch. For the aeipathia, use acupuncture on the shiny scalp. Only when the blood is purple, then hair will grow."

Feng's Secret Record (冯氏锦囊秘录 , *Féng Shì Jǐn Náng Mì Lù*)
"发乃血之余，焦枯者血不足也，忽然脱落，头皮作痒，须眉并落者，乃血热生风，风木摇动之象也。"

"Hair is the manifestation of blood. Hair becomes dry and withered because blood is deficient. The symptom of hair suddenly dropping, including the beard and eyebrow with an itchy scalp is the expression of wind caused by blood-heat and an unsteadiness of wind and wood."

Complete Book of Patterns and Treatments in External Medicine (外科证治全书 , *Wài Kē Zhèng zhì Quán Shū*)
"油风，俗称落发。头发干枯，成风脱落，皮红光亮，痒甚，由血燥有风所致。头发为血余，肾主发，脾主血，发落宜补脾肾，故妇人产后，脾肾大虚多患之。丹溪云：脉弦气弱，皮毛枯槁，头发脱落，黄芪建中汤主之。发脱落及脐下痛者，四君子汤加熟地黄、鹿角胶，每日清晨用醇酒化服三钱。至于外治方法虽多，而错节盘根，还当内治。"
一、白秃无发，用花椒四两，汇浸收瓷器内，盖好不泄气，日以搽之。
二、赤秃无发，用牛角、羊角烧灰等分，猪脂调敷。
三、病后发落，用猴姜、野蔷薇枝煎汁刷之。
四、发秃不生，用嫩枣树皮一把，斫一尺许，满插空瓷瓶内，勿令到底，上面以火烧之，则下面必有汁滴瓶内，先以热水洗头，后将此汁刷在秃处，即生发矣。

　　五、毛发黄赤，用羊矢烧灰，和腊猪油涂之，至发黑为止。

　　六、发槁不泽，用木瓜浸油梳头，或用胡麻油常涂之。梳须用黄杨木者佳。

　　七、年老发白，当拨出白发，以白蜜涂毛孔中，仍以梧子捣汁涂之，必生黑发。

"Glossy scalp wind is commonly known as hair dropping. The symptoms are dry and flaky hair, red and shiny scalp, itchiness induced by pathogenic wind and dry blood. Hair is the surplus of blood. Kidney governs hair and spleen governs blood, so we should tonify kidney and spleen for hair loss. Postpartum women whose kidney and spleen are deficient also often have alopecia areata. Zhu Dan-xi said that *Huáng Qí Jiàn Zhōng Tāng* (黄芪建中汤) treats a wiry pulse, deficient qi, withering hair and hair loss.

In cases of alopecia and pain below the umbilicus, use *Sì Jūn Zǐ Tāng* (四君子汤) with *shú dì huáng* (Radix Rehmanniae Praeparata) and *lù jiāo jiāo* (Colla Cornus Cervi). Take three *qian* with wine every morning. Although there are many kinds of external therapies, to treat the root, it is better to use an internal therapy.

In cases of white baldness, dip with four liang *huā jiāo* (Pericarpium Zanthoxyli) in porcelain. Tighten the container to prevent the air from leaking. Apply to the affected areas.

In cases of red baldness, burn oxhorn and goat horns into ash. Mix with pig fat and apply the mixture to the affected areas.

In cases of baldness following other illnesses, decoct *hóu jiāng* [*gǔ suì bǔ*] (Rhizoma Drynariae) and multiflora rose, and apply with the decoction.

In cases of no hair growth, cut the cortex of Chinese jujubes into the length of one *chi*. Place them in a bottle and be sure that the herbs do not go to the bottom of the bottle. Burn the top of the herbs and allow their juices to drop to the bottom. Wash the head with hot water, and then apply the juice to the affected areas. Hair will regrow.

In cases of yellow and red hair, burn sheep feces into ash, and mix it with pig fat. Apply the mixture on the hair until the hair turns black.

In cases of withered and yellow hair, dip fructus Chaenomelis in oil and brush the hair with it. Or frequently apply oleum sesami on the head. The boxwood comb is better for the health of the hair.

In cases of aged and white hair patients, pull out the white hair and apply white honey to the hair follicle. Grind *wú tóng zǐ* (Semen Firmianae) until there is juice from it. Apply this on the head and hair will regrow.

Discussion of Blood Patterns—Blood Stasis (血证论·瘀血, *Xuè Zhèng Lùn: Yū Xuè*)

"凡系离经之血，与养荣周身之血已睽绝而不合，瘀血在上焦，或发脱不生。"

"Blood circulating outside the vessels is different from blood that nourishes the body. Blood stasis in upper burner may cause alopecia.

Correction on Errors in Medical Classics—Category of Tōng Qiào Huó Xuè Tāng's Indication (医林改错·通窍活血汤所治之症目, *Yī Lín Gǎi Cuò: Tōng Qiào Huó Xuè Tāng Suǒ Zhì Zhī Zhèng Mù*)

"……头发脱落，各医书皆言伤血，不知皮里肉外血瘀，阻塞血络，新血不能养发，故发脱落。"

"Other doctors believe that damaged blood is the cause of alopecia. They do not realize that blood stasis beneath the skin and outside the muscle regions can also obstruct vessels. Fresh blood cannot nourish hair, and alopecia inevitably occurs."

MODERN RESEARCH

Clinical Research

1. Pattern Differentiation and Corresponding Treatment

Liu Hui-yun [1] believes that there are cases with combined excess and deficiency syndromes where deficiency is the root and excess is the branch. However, deficiency syndromes are more common. Treatments in general should be flexible and change as the syndromes transforms and changes. For emergency cases, principles for treating symptoms in excess conditions are clearing heat, soothing the liver, regulating qi, activating blood and eliminating blood stasis. For chronic diseases, principles for tonifying deficiency syndromes are nourishing qi, tonifying blood, warming the Yang, nourishing the kidney, invigorating the spleen and reinforcing the stomach. The concepts of holism and pattern differentiation in Chinese medicine assure that the internal organs can be balanced and regenerated. For internal therapy, Chinese medical theory is guided by the four diagnostic methods and eight principles.

There are six methods: (1) strengthening the spleen and replenishing qi for deficiency of spleen and stomach with *Shēn Líng Bái Zhú Powder* (参苓白术散), (2) tonifying qi and blood for deficiency of qi and blood with *Bā Zhēn Tāng* (八珍汤), (3) nourishing the liver and kidney for liver and kidney deficiency with *Modified Qī Bǎo Měi Rán* Pill (七宝美髯片), (4) clearing heat and nourishing yin for yang hyperactivity and yin deficiency with modified *Yǎng Yīn Qīng Fèi Tāng* (养阴清肺汤), (5) soothing liver and regulating qi for liver-qi stagnation with Modified *Xiao Yao* Powder, and (6) activating blood circulation and eliminating blood stasis for blood stasis in the hair follicles with *Modified Tōng Qiào Huó Xuè Tāng* (通窍活血汤).

Wu De-zhen [2] treated patients with blood deficiency and wind dryness using *Yǎng Xuè Shēng Fà* Capsule (养血生发胶囊): *shú dì huáng* (Radix Rehmanniae Praeparata), *dāng guī* (Radix Angelicae Sinensis), *qiāng huó* (Rhizoma et Radix Notopterygii), *mù guā* (Fructus Chaenomelis), *chuān xiōng* (Rhizoma Chuanxiong), *tiān má* (Rhizoma Gastrodiae), *zhì hé shǒu wū* (Radix Polygoni Multiflori Praeparata cum Succo Glycines Sotae), and *bái sháo* (Radix Paeoniae Alba). This prescription was taken twice every day and four capsules each time.

The alternative prescription would be *Bān Tū* Pill (斑秃片): *shú dì huáng* (Radix Rehmanniae Praeparata), *hé shǒu wū* (Radix Polygoni Multiflori), *dāng guī* (Radix Angelicae Sinensis), *dān shēn* (Radix et Rhizoma Salviae Miltiorrhizae), *shēng dì huáng* (Radix Rehmanniae), *bái sháo* (Radix Paeoniae Alba) and *qiāng huó* (Rhizoma et Radix Notopterygii). This prescription was taken twice every day and 9 grams each time.

For deficiency of the liver and kidney, use *Èr Zhì* Pill (二至片) or *Qī Bǎo Měi Rán* Pill (七宝美髯片) twice every day and 9 grams each time. In cases of qi stagnation and blood stasis, use *Jia Wei Xiao Yao* Pill twice every day and 6 gram each time, or *Dà Huáng Zhè Chóng* Pill (大黄蟅虫片) twice every day and 1-2 pills each time. In cases of qi and blood deficiency, use *Shí Quán Dà Bǔ* Pill (十全大补片) or *Bā Zhēn* Pill (八珍片) twice every day and 9 grams each time. The therapeutic course is one month. Take *Liù Wèi Dì Huáng* Pill (六味地黄片) after 2 courses twice every day and 8 pills each time for 1-2 months.

For the Chinese herbal topical applications, *Fà Fù Shēng* Liniment (发复生搽剂) (including minoxidil, chloral hydrate and decamethasone) is applied on the affected areas. Rub it on every morning and night until there is a hot sensation (without causing abrasions). The therapeutic course is one month, and it should be taken for four courses.

Of the 96 cases treated, 67 cases recovered and 20 were effective. The total effective rate was 95.8%.

2. Specific Formulas

Ruan Jin-feng [3] used oral tablets of Tripterygium Wilfordii (3.3 μg triptolide in each tablet). Two pills were taken each time, three times a day. Patients also used a topical application of 10% capsicum tincture twice every day for three months. Patients came in for a return visit every 15 days. They were also given follow-up surveys 3 months after therapy. Of the 44 cases treated, 20 cases were cured, 13 cases were effective, 10 cases improved and 1 case was not effective. The total recovery rate was 45.45% and the total effective rate was about 75%.

Results indicate that triprygium wilfordii polyglycosidium is a new immunity agent which is similar to the effects of hypothalamic corticotrophin, however it has different mechanisms without the side effects of hormone medications. Its influence on IL-2 is similar with cyclosporine, but its approach is completely different. Compared to other immunosuppressant drugs, its ability to focus more specifically on T cells and activate T cells is more appealing. It is useful in the clinical treatment of alopecia areata.

Zhou Ya [4] treated 94 cases with oral tablets of Tripterygium Wilfordii. Of all the 94 cases, 43 cases were cured, 22 cases were quite effective, and 12 cases were effective. The total effective rate was 77%.

Ma Jian-guo [5] used modified *Yì Gōng Sǎn* (益功散): *huáng qí* (Radix Astragali) 45g, *chén pí* (Pericarpium Citri Reticulatae) 6g, *gān cǎo* (Radix et Rhizoma Glycyrrhizae) 9g, *dǎng shēn* (Radix Codonopsis) 15g, *bái zhú* (Rhizoma Atractylodis Macrocephalae) 12g and *fú líng*(Poria) 12g. One decoction was taken per day. The decoction was taken 1 hour before every meal. The formula was also added to 1000ml of 50% alcohol and soaked for 1 week. The instructions were to use 70 ml of this liquid to 50% concentration of *Ban Mao* Tincture 30ml. Apply on the alopecia area twice every day.

Of the 50 cases treated, 41 were cured, 5 cases improved, and 1 case was invalid. The effective rate was 92%.

Gong Yi-yun [6] treated 126 cases with *Shēng Fà Tāng* (生发汤) for internal use and *Sheng Fa* Tincture for external use.

The ingredients of *Shēng Fà Tāng* are: *dāng guī* (Radix Angelicae Sinensis), *zhì hé shǒu wū* (Radix Polygoni Multiflori Praeparata cum Succo Glycines Sotae), *sāng shèn* (Fructus Mori), *nǔ zhēn zǐ* (Fructus Ligustri Lucidi) 12g, *mò hàn lián* (Herba Ecliptae) 12g, *yù jīn* (Radix Curcumae) 12g, *zhǐ qiào* (Fructus Aurantii) 12g, *huáng qí* (Radix Astragali) 15g, *dān shēn* (Radix et Rhizoma Salviae Miltiorrhizae) 15g, *yuǎn zhì* (Radix Polygalae) 9g, *sī guā luò* (Retinervus Luffae Fructus) 9g, and *shēng má* (Rhizoma Cimicifugae) 6g. The ingredients in *Shēng Fà* Tincture are *hé shǒu wū* (Radix Polygoni Multiflori) 200g, *bǔ gǔ zhī* (Fructus Psoraleae) 200g, *gān jiāng* (Rhizoma Zingiberis) 100g, *hóng huā* (Flos Carthami) 100g, *chuān xiōng* (Rhizoma Chuanxiong) 100g, *guì zhī* (Ramulus Cinnamomi) 100g, and *shé chuáng zǐ* (Fructus Cnidii) 100g. All of the herbs are cut and dipped into 3000ml of 75% concentration of alcohol for 10 days before draining out its the liquid.

The effective rate was as high as 99.20% after 3 months of topical application.

He Liang-xin [7] soaked six *bān máo* (Mylabris) in 100ml of 95% concentration of alcohol. The bottle was covered for 5 to 7 days. The tincture was applied on the affected areas 2-3 times everyday. One course of treatment was 15 days. Most patients had 2-3 courses with 5 courses as the maximum.

Of the 64 cases treated, 48 cases were cured (75%), 12 cases were effectual (18.8%), and 4 cases were effective (6.2%).

Chen Xun-jun [8] dipped *shēng jiāng* (Rhizoma Zingiberis Recens) into *Dān Hóng* Tincture (丹红酊) and applied it on the alopecia areas. The herbs of *Dān Hóng* Tincture are *hóng là jiāo* (paprika), *hóng huā* (Flos

Carthami), *huā jiāo* (Pericarpium Zanthoxyli), *dān shēn* (Radix et Rhizoma Salviae Miltiorrhizae), and *zhāng nǎo* (camenthol). The tincture was applied on the alopecia areas until the skin became red and hot. Apply 3-4 times every day. Patients also took cystine and vitamin B6 internally.

Of the 38 cases treated, 28 cases were cured which is 2% higher than the control group of minoxidil.

Chen Zhan-xue [9] prepared a tincture by grinding *fù zǐ* (Radix Aconiti Lateralis Praeparata) 20g, *gǔ suì bǔ* (Rhizoma Drynariae) 15g, and *cè bǎi yè* (Cacumen Platycladi) 25g into powder. Soak the powder into 60g of vinegar for 10 days. Dip sterilized cotton into the liquid and apply onto the alopecia areas at least 3 times a day, every day. Of the 22 cases treated, 7 patients grew sparse hair in the local area after 10 days of treatment. The new hair was the same as the surrounding hairs in color and thickness. Ten cases grew bushy and slightly yellow hair in the local area and the new hair became normal after a month. Three cases gradually grew bushy, and slightly yellow hair after 15 days and the new hair became normal after 40 days. Two cases were invalid after 30 days of treatment.

The total effective rate was 90.91%.

Zhao Yi-en [10] used *Sāng Chǔ Shēng Fà Tāng* (桑楮生发汤): *sāng shèn* (Fructus Mori) 30g, *chǔ shí zǐ* (Fructus Broussonetiae) 30g, *huáng qí* (Radix Astragali) 30g, *shú dì huáng* (Radix Rehmanniae Praeparata) 12g, *dāng guī* (Radix Angelicae Sinensis) 12g, *zhì hé shǒu wū* (Radix Polygoni Multiflori Praeparata cum Succo Glycines Sotae) 12g, *dǎng shēn* (Radix Codonopsis) 12g, *bái zhú* (Rhizoma Atractylodis Macrocephalae) 12g, *fú líng* (Poria) 12g, *yuǎn zhì* (Radix Polygalae) 10g, *ròu guì* (Cortex Cinnamomi), *tiān má* (Rhizoma Gastrodiae) 10g, *chén pí* (Pericarpium Citri Reticulatae) 10g, *wǔ wèi zǐ* (Fructus Schisandrae Chinensis) 6g, and *zhì gān cǎo* (Radix et Rhizoma Glycyrrhizae Praeparata cum Melle) 6g. Decoct the herbs over a low flame for 20 minutes and pour out the liquid. Then decoct them again in the same manner. Mix the three bottles of the liquid and take it 5 times, about 200 ml each time and three times daily. Use *shēng jiāng* (Rhizoma Zingiberis Recens) to rub the alopecia areas. The decoction was generally taken for 1 month or 2-3 months for patients with severe conditions.

Of the 36 cases treated, 30 cases were cured and 6 cases were effectual. The curative rate was 83.3% and effective rate was 100%.

Zhou Cong-he [11] used *Bǔ Shèn Yǎng Xuè Capsule* (补肾养血胶囊): *zhì hé shǒu wū* (Radix Polygoni Multiflori Praeparata cum Succo Glycines Sotae), *shú dì huáng* (Radix Rehmanniae Praeparata), *fú líng* (Poria), *dāng guī* (Radix Angelicae Sinensis), *gǒu qǐ zǐ* (Fructus Lycii) for internal medicine. For external treatment, he used *Bǔ Gǔ Zhī* Tincture (补骨脂酊): *bǔ gǔ zhī* (Fructus Psoraleae), *hóng huā* (Flos Carthami), *bái zhǐ* (Radix Angelicae Dahuricae) and *xì xīn* (Radix et Rhizoma Asari). All herbs were soaked in 75% concentration of alcohol.

Of the 91 cases treated, 60 cases were cured, 17 cases were effectual, and 10 cases improved. The total effective rate was 95.6%.

Yang Shu-cheng [12] treated 32 cases with *Shēng Fà Tāng* (生发汤): *hé shǒu wū* (Radix Polygoni Multiflori) 30g, *rén shēn* (Radix Ginseng) (stewed) 15g, *zhì huáng qí* (Radix Astragali Praeparata cum Melle) 15g, *bái sháo* (Radix Paeoniae Alba) 15g, *qín pí* (Cortex Fraxini) 15g, *dāng guī* (Radix Angelicae Sinensis) 15g, *dān shēn* (Radix et Rhizoma Salviae Miltiorrhizae) 12g, *bái zhú* (Rhizoma Atractylodis Macrocephalae) 10g, *chái hú* (Radix Bupleuri) 10g, *chuān xiōng* (Rhizoma Chuanxiong) 10g, *wú gōng* (Scolopendra) 1 piece (swallowed), and *gān cǎo* (Radix et Rhizoma Glycyrrhizae) 5g. All the herbs were decocted and taken three times a day. A prescription was finished in two days. *Shēng Fà* Cream (生发膏) included *cǎo wū* (Radix Aconiti Kusnezoffii) powder mixed with *shēng jiāng* (Rhizoma Zingiberis Recens) juice into paste. The paste was applied on the affected areas once daily.

The total curative rate was 96.87%.

Lu Guang-long [13] used *Shēng Fà Tāng* (生发汤): *shēng dì huáng* (Radix Rehmanniae) 15g, *shú dì huáng* (Radix Rehmanniae Praeparata) 15g, *gǒu qǐ zǐ* (Fructus Lycii) 15g, *zhì hé shǒu wū* (Radix Polygoni Multiflori Praeparata cum Succo Glycines Sotae) 15g, *mò hàn lián* (Herba Ecliptae) 10g, *nǚ zhēn zǐ* (Fructus Ligustri Lucidi) 10g, *tiān má* (Rhizoma Gastrodiae) 10g, *jí lí* (Fructus Tribuli) 10g, *cè bǎi yè* (Cacumen Platycladi) 10g, *tù sī zǐ* (Semen Cuscutae) 10g, *chuān xiōng* (Rhizoma Chuanxiong) 6g, and *jú huā* (Flos Chrysanthemi) 6g. One dose per day. Drink the decoction in the morning and night. For external application, he used *Bān Máo Tāng* (斑蝥汤): *bān máo* (Mylabris) 8 pc., *máo jiāng [gǔ suì bǔ]* (Rhizoma Drynariae) 15g, and *dōng chóng xià cǎo* (Cordyceps) 15g. Soak these herbs in 200ml of alcohol for 15 days. Shake the bottle frequently. Apply the tincture on alopecia areas 3-4 times daily.

Of the 32 cases treated, the effective rate was 100%.

Long Chang-da [14] gave internal medicine using *Guī Wū Mixture* (归乌合剂): *dāng guī* (Radix Angelicae Sinensis), *zhì hé shǒu wū* (Radix Polygoni Multiflori Praeparata cum Succo Glycines Sotae), *nǚ zhēn zǐ* (Fructus Ligustri Lucidi), *huáng qí* (Radix Astragali). Of the 60 cases treated, the total marked effective rate was 68.3% and the total effective rate was 88.3%. The hair pulling test measured how easily hair fell out. Comparing before and after treatment, the hair pulling test rating from positive to negative was 89.1%, which indicated that the herbal mixture effectively controlled alopecia.

Ma Hai-ping [15] used a self-made decoction, *Shēng Fà Tāng* (生发汤): *hé shǒu wū* (Radix Polygoni Multiflori) 15g, *shú dì huáng* (Radix Rehmanniae Praeparata) 18g, *hēi zhī ma* (Semen Sesami Nigrum) 30g, *bái sháo* (Radix Paeoniae Alba) 30g, *chuān xiōng* (Rhizoma Chuanxiong), *shān zhū yú* (Fructus Corni) 15g, *gǒu qǐ zǐ* (Fructus Lycii) 15g, *tù sī zǐ* (Semen Cuscutae) 15g, and *qiāng huó* (Rhizoma et Radix Notopterygii) 6g.

Seventy-two cases were treated. In cases of blood heat, add *shēng dì* (Radix Rehmanniae Recens) 15g and *mǔ dān pí* (Cortex Moutan) 12g. In cases of liver-qi stagnation, add *xiāng fù* (Rhizoma Cyperi) 12g and *yù jīn* (Radix Curcumae) 15g. In cases of significant kidney deficiency, add *lù jiǎo jiāo* (Colla Cornus Cervi) (melted by heat) and *sāng shèn* (Fructus Mori) 15g. In cases of insomnia, add *hé huān huā* (Flos Albiziae) 15g and *shǒu wū téng* (Caulis Polygoni Multiflori) 30g. The course of treatment was one month. Two courses of treatment were recommended.

Of the 46 cases were treated, 8 cases were effectual and 2 cases were invalid. The total effective rate was 97.2%.

Zhang Jin-hua [16] created self-made formulas, *Shēng Fà Tāng* (生发汤) and *Shēng Fà* Tincture, to treat 47 cases. Fresh *cè bǎi yè* (Cacumen Platycladi) was soaked in 75% concentration of alcohol for 30 days. After filtering out the liquid, add 1.5% *nào yáng huā* (Flos Rhododendri Mollis) and an appropriate amount of *rén shēn* (Radix et Rhizoma Ginseng) and *lú huì* (Aloe). Keep the container sealed for 30 days. Then filter out the liquid and divide it into parts of 60ml and keep them in separate plastic bottles. Dip a piece of *shēng jiāng* (Rhizoma Zingiberis Recens) into the liquid and rub it on alopecia areas 2-3 times daily.

His internal medicine was *Shēng Fà Tāng: zhì hé shǒu wū* (Radix Polygoni Multiflori Praeparata cum Succo Glycines Sotae) 30g, *fú líng* (Poria) 15g, *huái niú xī* (Radix Achyranthis Bidentatae) 15g, *dāng guī* (Radix Angelicae Sinensis) 15g, *gǒu qǐ zǐ* (Fructus Lycii) 15g, *bǔ gǔ zhī* (Fructus Psoraleae) 15g, *tù sī zǐ* (Semen Cuscutae) 15g, *shēng dì* (Radix Rehmanniae) 15g, *dān shēn* (Radix et Rhizoma Salviae Miltiorrhizae) 15g, *chuān xiōng* (Rhizoma Chuanxiong) 8g, and *zé xiè* (Rhizoma Alismatis) 15g.

In cases of qi and blood deficiency, add *huáng qí* (Radix Astragali) 20g and *dǎng shēn* (Radix Codonopsis) 15g. In cases of liver and kidney deficiency, sore and aching low back and knees, add *xiān máo* (Rhizoma

Curculiginis) 15g and *yín yáng huò* (Herba Epimedii) 15g. In cases of melancholy and sleeping problems, add *fú shén* (Sclerotium Poriae Cocos Paradicis) 15g, *suān zǎo rén* (Semen Ziziphi Spinosae) 10g, and *shǒu wū téng* (Caulis Polygoni Multiflori) 15g. In cases of oily hair, add *jiāo shān zhā* (Fructus Crataegi Praeparatus) 30g and *jué míng zǐ* (Semen Cassiae) 15g. The course of treatment was 15 days. Therapeutic results were found generally after 3 courses of treatment.

Thirty cases were cured, 10 cases were significantly effective, and 5 cases were effective. The total effective rate was 95.74%.

Yang Shi-zhong [17] combined internal and external therapy.

He used *Jiā Wèi Sì Wù Tāng* (加味四物汤) for internal therapy: *dāng guī* (Radix Angelicae Sinensis) 15g, *bái sháo* (Radix Paeoniae Alba) 15g, *chì sháo* (Radix Paeoniae Rubra) 15g, *shēng dì huáng* (Radix Rehmanniae) 15g, *shú dì huáng* (Radix Rehmanniae Praeparata) 15g, *chuān xiōng* (Rhizoma Chuanxiong) 15g, *dān shēn* (Radix et Rhizoma Salviae Miltiorrhizae) 15g, and *hé shǒu wū* (Radix Polygoni Multiflori) 15g. Take one prescription daily. Decoct and take every morning and evening.

Bǔ Gǔ Zhī Tincture (补骨脂酊) was the external therapy. Soak *bǔ gǔ zhī* (Fructus Psoraleae) 150g in 500ml of 75% alcohol for one week. Apply the tincture on alopecia once daily for 2 months.

Of the 57 cases treated, there were 8 cases of alopecia totalis. The total effective rate was 91.33%.

Xie Xun-hui [18] used *Bǔ Shèn Yǎng Xuè* Pill (补肾养血片): *hé shǒu wū* (Radix Polygoni Multiflori) 240g, *shú dì* (Radix Rehmanniae Praeparata) 60g, *dāng guī* (Radix Angelicae Sinensis) 90g, *chuān xiōng* (Rhizoma Chuanxiong) 20g, *dān shēn* (Radix et Rhizoma Salviae Miltiorrhizae) 90g, *jiāng huó* (Angelica sylvestris) 20g, *cè bǎi yè* (Cacumen Platycladi) 90g, *nǚ zhēn zǐ* (Fructus Ligustri Lucidi) 60g and *mò hàn lián* (Herba Ecliptae) 60g. All the herbs were grinded into powder and rolled into honey balls (6g per ball) for oral intake.

His external therapy was *Bǔ Shèn Huó Xuè Shēng Fà Jīng* (补肾活血生发精): *hóng shēn* (Radix et Rhizoma Ginseng Rubra) 100g, *huáng qí* (Radix Astragali) 200g, *dāng guī* (Radix Angelicae Sinensis) 60g, *chuān xiōng* (Rhizoma Chuanxiong) 60g, *gān jiāng* (Rhizoma Zingiberis) 60g, *táo rén* (Semen Persicae) 60g, *hóng huā* (Flos Carthami) 50g, *dān shēn* (Radix et Rhizoma Salviae Miltiorrhizae) 100g and *bǔ gǔ zhī* (Fructus Psoraleae) 100g. All herbs were soaked in 2000ml of kaoliang spirit (liquor) for 2 weeks. Mix the spirit with 1% minoxidil at equal proportions of 50/50.

Of the 56 cases treated, 42 cases were cured and 11 cases were markedly effective. The total effective rate was 94.6%.

Chen Su [19] used *Fà Bǎo* Instant Granules (发宝冲剂): *dāng guī* (Radix Angelicae Sinensis) 15g, *gǒu qǐ zǐ* (Fructus Lycii) 15g, *suān zǎo rén* (Semen Ziziphi Spinosae) 15g, *yuǎn zhì* (Radix Polygalae) 15g, *hé shǒu wū* (Radix Polygoni Multiflori) 30g, *sāng shèn* (Fructus Mori) 30g, *hēi zhī ma* (Semen Sesami Nigrum) 30g, *hé táo rén* (Semen Juglandis) 30g, and *cè bǎi yè* (Cacumen Platycladi) 30g.

The external treatment was *Shēng Fà* Tincture (生发酊): *hóng huā* (Flos Carthami) 60g, *gān jiāng* (Rhizoma Zingiberis) 90g, *dāng guī* (Radix Angelicae Sinensis), *chì sháo* (Radix Paeoniae Rubra) 100g, *shēng dì* (Radix Rehmanniae) 100g, and *cè bǎi yè* (Cacumen Platycladi) 100g. All the herbs were soaked in 60% alcohol for 10 days.

Of the 62 cases treated, 51 cases were cured, 7 cases were markedly effectual, and 3 cases were effective. The total effective rate was 98.4%.

Deng Hai-qing [20] used *Yǎng Xuè Shēng Fà Tāng* (养血生发汤): *huáng qí* (Radix Astragali) 30g, *shú dì* (Radix Rehmanniae Praeparata) 15g, *bái zhú* (Rhizoma Atractylodis Macrocephalae) 15g, *bái sháo* (Radix Paeoniae Alba) 15g, *shǒu wū téng* (Caulis Polygoni Multiflori) 15g, *tiān má* (Rhizoma Gastrodiae) 6g, *mù guā* (Fructus Chaenomelis) 6g, *dōng chóng xià cǎo* (Cordyceps) 6g, *dāng guī* (Radix Angelicae Sinensis) 10g., *chuān xiōng*

(Rhizoma Chuanxiong) 10g, *zhì yuǎn zhì* (Radix Polygalae Praeparata) 10g, *hóng huā* (Flos Carthami) 9g, *mò hàn lián* (Herba Ecliptae) 9g, *nǚ zhēn zǐ* (Fructus Ligustri Lucidi) 9g. Decoct the herbs and take one dosage prescription daily.

The external therapy was *Bǎi Yè Shēng Fà* Tincture (柏叶生发酊): *hóng huā* (Flos Carthami) 9g, *gān jiāng* (Rhizoma Zingiberis) 12g, *chì sháo* (Radix Paeoniae Rubra) 13g, *dāng guī* (Radix Angelicae Sinensis) 18g, *shēng dì huáng* (Radix Rehmanniae) 18g, and *cè bǎi yè* (Cacumen Platycladi) 18g. Cut the herbs and soak them into 500ml of 75% concentration of alcohol. Seal the container for 10 days. Shake the container twice daily. After 10 days, open the container and apply an appropriate amount of liquid to the alopecia areas 3 times a day. One course of treatment is one month. Improvements were observed after 2 courses of treatment.

Of the 46 cases treated, 31 cases recovered, 10 cases were markedly effectual, and 4 cases were effective. The total effective rate was 97.8%.

3. Acupuncture and Moxibustion

Bai Guang-ping [21] used a head and neck traction belt and plum-blossom needle therapy on alopecia areas for 97 cases of alopecia areata with good results. Patients were treated with cervical and occipital traction belt for 30 minutes. The level of intensity and traction varied to each patient's comfort level. After traction, the areas of alopecia were cleaned with 2.5% iodine, and then cleaned with 75% concentration of alcohol. Mild tapping induced slight bleeding. The blood was left unwiped. In most cases, new hair grew after 3 weeks of traction treatment and 10 treatments of tapping. For a few critical alopecia areata patients, if new hair barely grew out, traction was done for 2 more weeks. He performed heavy tapping on the alopecia areas every two days to induce more bleeding. After bleeding, he did not close the acupuncture point opening nor clean the blood. After 3 weeks of continuous treatments for

97 cases, soft, thin and delicate hair began to grow. After 4-5 weeks of treatment, hair became more abundant and stronger. After 5-6 weeks of treatment, patients' hair became normal and healthy. Clinical follow ups were conducted for 1 year and for cases of relapse.

Ma Ji-mei [22] used dermal needles and Chinese medicine together to treat 32 cases. Alopecia areas were cleaned with 75% concentration of alcohol before mild tapping with pyonex. Local skin became slightly flushed and red, but there was no pain for the patients. Tapping was done on a daily basis. Fresh *shēng jiāng* (Rhizoma Zingiberis Recens) was applied on alopecia areas every night before sleeping. It is pungent, warm, and dispersing. *Zhì hé shǒu wū* (Radix Polygoni Multiflori Praeparata cum Succo Glycines Sotae) 30g was decocted and its liquor was taken every 100ml. Of the 32 cases treated, 28 cases were cured and 3 cases improved. The author believes that *zhì hé shǒu wū* (Radix Polygoni Multiflori Praeparata cum Succo Glycines Sotae) tonifies the liver and kidney and nourishes the essence and blood. Both the tapping and herbal decoction proved to be effective treatments.

Sheng Ming-ying [23] used seven-star needle therapy and a topical herbal application to treat alopecia areata. The herbs in *Kè Tū Níng Dīng* (克秃宁酊) are: *gāo lì shēn* (korean ginseng) 30g, *hé shǒu wū* (Radix Polygoni Multiflori) 150g, *gǔ suì bǔ* (Rhizoma Drynariae) 150g, *mò hàn lián* (Herba Ecliptae) 150g, and *hóng huā* (Flos Carthami) 50g. Grind the herbs into powder. Mix the powder, slices of *shēng jiāng* (Rhizoma Zingiberis Recens) 50g and fresh *cè bǎi yè* (Cacumen Platycladi) 400g. Soak them into 1000ml of 95% alcohol into a tightly sealed bottle for half a month. Then drain the liquid and apply it on the affected areas. Twenty-eight cases were treated. After 2 weeks of treatment, vellus hair grew and the hair became thick and black after 4 weeks of treatment. The color and density of the new hair resumed their normal structure. All patients recovered after 4 to 8 weeks of treatment.

Experimental Studies

1. Research on the Efficacy of Herbal Prescriptions

1) Xu Qian [24] used blood viscosity as a measurement for 56 alopecia areata cases measured by 6 rheology indicators. Patients were divided into groups for the active stage or resting stage. Patients were also assigned to groups based on Chinese medicine syndromes, deficiency and excess groups. These groups were compared to a control of group of 35 individuals without alopecia areata. The researchers used t-test statistical analysis to analyze the results.

Compared with the control group, the experimental groups showed significant increase in the reduced viscosity at high shear of whole blood, viscosity at low shear, hematocrit, high-performance liquid chromatography, as well as significant reduction in and aggregate degree of erythrocyte ($p<0.05$). The rising of plasma viscosity was not shown to be statistically significant. Compared with the control group, the active stage group showed significant differences in the 6 indicators ($p<0.05$). The resting stage group showed significant difference in reduced viscosity at low shear, hematocrit and high-performance liquid chromatography ($p<0.05$). All 6 indicators of 35 patients in the excess syndrome stage showed significant difference ($p<0.05$). The deficiency group showed significant difference in reduced viscosity at low shear, hematocrit, high-performance liquid chromatography, and aggregate degree of erythrocyte ($p<0.05$). There were significant changes in the rheology indicators for patients with alopecia areata. Increased blood viscosity and impairment of microcirculation offers deeper insight into the alopecia areata's pathogenesis, which would change along with disease stages and its severity. It is also implied that invigorating blood and resolving stasis could improve clinical outcomes.

2) Lil Luo-en [25] proved through experimental studies that pachymaran significantly improves lab animals' peritoneal macrophage phagocytosis, activates the T cells and B cells, and enhances immune function. The method was to grind *fú líng* (Poria) 500-1000g into powder. Six grams were given orally twice a day with boiled water. The alternate option was to decoct *fú líng* (Poria) 10g with *bǔ gǔ zhī* (Fructus Psoraleae) 25g and *mò hàn lián* (Herba Ecliptae) 25g before bedtime.

3) Treatment for alopecia commonly includes the herb, *hé shǒu wū* (Radix Polygoni Multiflori), which contains 3.7% lecithin. Lecithin plays a significant role in the function of nerve tissue, especially the brain and spinal cord. Lecithin is also an important component of cell membranes and cellular growth and development. *Hé shǒu wū* (Radix Polygoni Multiflori) supports the internal pharmacological dynamics for tonifying the Liver and Kidney, and nourishing essence and blood.[26]

2. Research on the Efficacy of Herbal Prescriptions

1) Chen Da-can [27] used an internal medicine formula named *Yì Fà Zhì Jì A* (益发制剂 A): *zhì hé shǒu wū* (Radix Polygoni Multiflori Praeparata cum Succo Glycines Sotae), *nǚ zhēn zǐ* (Fructus Ligustri Lucidi), *huáng qí* (Radix Astragali), *shān zhā* (Fructus Crataegi), *pú gōng yīng* (Herba Taraxaci), *jī xuě cǎo* (Herba Centellae), and *gān cǎo* (Radix et Rhizoma Glycyrrhizae). For the external therapy, he used *Yì FàZhì Jì B* Tincture (益发制剂 B 外用酊): *zhì cì wǔ jiā* (Radix et Rhizoma seu Caulis Acanthopanacis Senticosi Praeparata), *rén shēn yè* (Folium Ginseng), *huā jiāo* (Pericarpium Zanthoxyli), *cè bǎi yè* (Cacumen Platycladi), *chuān xiōng* (Rhizoma Chuanxiong) and *bīng piàn* (Borneolum Syntheticum).

Three hundred and nineteen patients with alopecia were treated in a randomized, single-blinded, controlled trial using *Yì Fà Zhì Jì A*. Of the 310 cases, 205 cases were cured, 63 cases were markedly effective, and 37 cases were effective. The results showed that *Yì Fà Zhì Jì A* had a total effective rate of 95.6%, significantly higher than that of the control group with the western medication, mechlorethamine tincture. Experiments revealed that *Yì Fà Zhì Jì* could regulate T lymphocytes and its distribution, increase the level of serum interleukin-2, and strengthen immunological function in patients.

2) Ma Bo-ping [28] used *Shēng Fà Líng* Tincture (生发灵酊): *dāng guī* (Radix Angelicae Sinensis), *xī hóng huā* (Stigma Croci), *cè bǎi yè* (Cacumen Platycladi), *hé shǒu wū* (Radix Polygoni Multiflori), *shēng dì huáng* (Radix Rehmanniae), *chì sháo* (Radix Paeoniae Rubra), and *gān jiāng* (Rhizoma Zingiberis) for external use. Of the 280 cases treated, 171 were cured and 92 cases improved. The total effective rate was 93.9%, which was higher than the minoxidil control group. After treatment, the Tumor Necrosis Factor decreased, while ANA, anti mitochondrial antibody and reactive antibody of the heart turned negative, indicating that the tincture could enhance immune function. It also suggested that the tincture could reduce a positive rate of auto antibodies accordingly in order to treat alopecia areata caused by autoimmune disorders.

3) Lin Rui-fen [29] treated with *Sān Téng* Instant Granules (三藤冲剂): *leé gōng téng* (Tripterygium wilfkrdii Hook) 10g, *shǒu wū téng* (Caulis Polygoni Multiflori) 20g, *jī xuè téng* (Caulis Spatholobi) 20g, and *gān cǎo* (Radix et Rhizoma Glycyrrhizae) 3g. The herbs were decocted for oral intake, three times a day. The course of treatment was 20 days. Of the 30 cases treated, the curative rate was 53.3% and the effective rate was 93.3%. The markers, CD3, CD4 and CD8, increased while the ratio of CD4 to CD8 decreased, indicating that the granules improved the patients' imbalanced immune functions. No toxins or deleterious effect were found in the dosage amounts. The granules were also inexpensive treatments for alopecia areata.

4) Wan Ke-ying [30] observed the clinical effects of *Qǐ Jú Dì Huáng* Bolus (杞菊地黄丸) on alopecia areacta, and measured the microelement

content in the hair of the patients before and after treatment. The results showed that patients' iron, zinc and copper were initially lower than normal, however they increased after the treatment. It suggested that *Qǐ Jú Dì Huáng* Bolus could improve the clinical efficacy of alopecia areacta patients, possibly by its effects on the metabolism of microelements in the patients.

REFERENCES

[1] Liu Hui-yun. Six Internal Therapies on Alopecia Areata (论内治斑秃六法). *Journal of Traditional Chinese Medicine* (光明中医), 2004, l9(4); 3l-32

[2] Wu De-zheng, Liu Shi-feng, Yue Yong-huai. Clinical Observations of Combined Chinese Medicine and Biomedicine on 96 Alopecia Areata Patients. (中西医结合治疗斑秃96例临床观察) *Hebei Journal of Traditional Chinese Medicine* (河北中医), 2005,27(6): 444-445

[3] Ruan Jin-feng. Clinical Observation on 44 Alopecia Areata Patients Treated by Tablets of Tripterygium Wilfordii (雷公藤片治疗斑秃44例临床疗效观察). *Journal of Qiqihar Medical College* (齐齐哈尔医学院学报) 2004, 25(6):627-628

[4] Zhou Ya, Fan Xiu-zhi, Yao Chun-lin, et al. Clinical Observation of 94 Alopecia Areata Patients Treated by Tablets of Tripterygium Wilfordii (雷公藤片治疗94例斑秃疗效观察). *New Chinese Medicine* (新医学), 2000, 31(3): 164

[5] Ma Jian-guo. Clinical Observation of Modified Yi Gong Powder on 50 Alopecia Areata Patients (异功散加味治疗斑秃50例疗效观察). *Hebei Journal of Traditional Chinese Medicine* (河北中医), 1998,20(1)37

[6] Gong Yi-yun. *Sheng Fa Tang* for Internal Therapy and *Sheng Fa Dīng* for External Therapy on 126 Alopecia Areata Patients (内服生发饮外用生发酊治疗斑秃126例). *Yun Nan Journal of Traditional Chinese Medicine* (云南中医药杂志), 1997,18(4): 14

[7] He Liang-xin. *Treating 64 Alopecia Areata Patients with Cantharides Tincture* (斑蝥酊治疗斑秃64例). *Modern Journal of Integrated Traditional Chinese and Western Medicine* (中华现代中西医结合). 2004, 4(12): 330-231

[8] Chen Xun-jun. *Dan Hong Dīng* on 38 Alopecia Areata Patients (丹红酊治疗斑秃38例). *Herald of Medicine* (医药导报) 2003, 22(1): 50

[9] Chen Zhan-xue. Chinese Drugs' Vinegar on Alopecia Areata (中药醋浸液治疗斑秃). *Journal of External Therapy of Traditional Chinese Medicine* (中医外治杂志), 2004,13(1): 45

[10] Zhao Yi-en, Zhao Zeen. *Sang Chu Sheng Fa Tang* on 36 Alopecia Areata Patients (桑楮生发汤治疗斑秃36例). *Journal of Sichuan Traditional Chinese Medicine* (四川中医). 2004, 22(1): 82

[11] Zhou Cong-he. Clinical Observation of Bu Sheng Yang Xue Capsule on 91 Alopecia Areata Patients (补肾养血胶囊治疗斑秃91例临床观察). *New Chinese Medicine* (新中医), 2002, 34(1): 26

[12] Yang Shu-cheng. Chinese Medicine for Internal and External Therapies on 32 Alopecia Areata Patients (中药内外合用治疗斑秃32例). *Journal of Sichuan Traditional Chinese Medicine* (四川中医). 1998, 16(5): 45

[13] Lu Guang-long, Zhu Chuan-xiu. *Sheng Fa Tang* for Internal Therapy and Ban Ao Wine for External Application on 32 Alopecia Areata Patients (生发汤等内服斑蝥酒外涂治疗斑秃32例). *Journal of Anhui Traditional Chinese Medical College* (安徽中医学院学报), 1997, 16(1): 32

[14] Long Da-chang, Zhang Jia-lin, Li Shao-xing, et al. Clinical Observation of Chinese Medicine Gui Wu Mixture on Alopecia Areata (中药归乌合剂治疗斑秃疗效观察). *Chinese Journal of Dermatology* (中华皮肤科杂志), 2000, 33(2): 130

[15] Ma Hai-ping. Self-made *Sheng Fa Tang* on 72 Alopecia Areata Patients (自制生发饮治疗斑秃72例). *China's Naturopathy* (中国民间疗法), 2005, 13(1O): 35-36

[16] Zhang Jin-hua, Zhang Xi-jun. Self-made *Sheng Fa Tang* and *Sheng Fa Dīng* on Alopecia Areata Patients (自拟生发汤合生发酊治疗斑秃47例). *Journal of External Therapy of Traditional Chinese Medicine* (中医外治杂志), 2004, 13(5): 6-7

[17] Yang Shi-zhong, Fang Zhuo. Chinese Medicine on 57 Alopecia Areata Patients (中医药治疗斑秃57例). *Jilin Journal of Traditional Chinese Medicine* (吉林中医药), 1996, (2): 14

[18] Xie Xun-hui, Chen Chang-peng. Clinical Observation of Bu Shen Yang Xue Sheng Fa Bolus on 57 Alopecia Areata Patients (补肾养血生发丸治疗斑秃56例疗效观察). *Southern China Journal of Dermato-Venereology* (岭南皮肤性病科杂志), 2003, 10(2): 85

[19] Chen Su. Fa Bao Instant Granules Combined with *Sheng Fa Dīng* on 62 Alopecia Areata Patients (发宝冲剂配合生发酊治疗斑秃62例). *Journal of Practical Traditional Chinese Medicine* (实用中医药杂志), 2002, 18(9): 17

[20] Deng Hai-qing, Pan Chao-xia. Clinical Research of *Yang Xue Sheng Fa Tang* Combined with *Bai Ye Sheng Fa Dīng* on 46 Alopecia Areata Patients (养血生发汤配合柏叶生发酊治疗斑秃46例疗效观察). *New Chinese Medicine*(新中医). 2004, 36(5): 46-47

[21] Bai Guang-ping. Cervical and Occipital Belt Traction and Plum-Blossom Needle Therapy on Alopecia Areata (颈椎牵引加梅花针叩刺治疗斑秃). *Practical Journal of Rural Doctor*(中国实用乡村医生杂志), 2005,12(4): 27

[22] Ma Ji-mei, Zhao Jia-yi. Therapeutic Effect of Dermal Needle and Chinese Medicine on Refractory Alopecia Areata (皮肤针配合中药治疗难治性斑秃32例疗效观察). *The Medical Journal of Industrial Enterprise* (工企医刊). 2001;14 (5):57

[23] Shen Ming-ying, Han Tao. Seven-star Needle Combine with Ke Tu Ning Tincture for External Application on Alopecia Areata (七星针叩击加克秃宁酊外擦治疗斑秃). *Journal of External Therapy of Traditional Chinese Medicine* (中医外治杂志), 2001,10(3):37

[24] Xu Qian，Shi Wei-min，Shen Liang-liang. The Relationship of TCM Grouping and Disturbance of Microcirculation in 56 Cases of Alopecia areata (斑秃的中医辨证分型与微循环障碍临床56例). *Journal of Tongji University* (*Medical Science*) (同济大学学报(医学版)) 2005, 26 (2): 65-66

[25] Li Luo-en, et al. Mechanism and New Clinical Application of Fú Ling (Poria) (茯苓的药理及临床新用). *Primary Journal of Chinese Materia Medica* (基层中药杂志), 1997,11(3): 55

[26] Yang Ji, Ji Shao-liang, Ji Chun-ru. Guidelines for Compatibility and Application on Clinical Symptoms (临证用药配伍指南). *First Edition.Beijing: The Medicine Science and Technology Press of China* (第一版.北京:中国医药科技出版社) 1996: 112

[27] Chen Da-can, Xuan Guo-wei, Hu Dong-liu, et al. Treatment of Alopecia Areata with Yifa Oral Liquid: A Clinical Observation of 319 Patients (中药益发制剂治疗斑秃319例临床观察). *Journal of Guangzhou University of Traditional Chinese Medicine* (广州中医药大学学报) 1996, 13 (3, 4): 41-43

[28] Ma Ping-bo. *Sheng Fa Ling Dīng* on 280 Alopecia Areata Patients (生发灵酊治疗斑秃280例). *Herald of Medicine.*(医药导报), 2003, 22(6): 385

[29] Lin Rui-fen. Clinical and Immunological Research of San Teng Instant Granules on Alopecia Areata (三藤冲剂治疗斑秃的临床与免疫学研究). *Journal of Fujian College of Traditional Chinese Medicine* (福建中医学院学报). 2004, 14 (5): 7-8

[30] Wan Ke-ying, Li Chao-hua, Luo Li-fang. Clinical Observations on Treating Alopecia Areata by Qi Ju Di Huang Bolus and Change about Microelement (杞菊地黄丸治疗斑秃的临床观察及微量元素的变化). *Chinese Journal of the Practical Chinese With Modern Medicine* (中华实用中西医杂志), 2004, 4(1): 2168-2169

Androgenetic Alopecia

by

Fan Rui-qiang
Chief Physician & Professor of Chinese External Medicine

Hu Dong-liu, M.S. TCM
Associate Chief Physician of Chinese External Medicine

Xuan Guo-wei
Chief Physician & Professor of Chinese External Medicine

Chen Xiu-yang, M.S. TCM
Attending Physician of Chinese External Medicine

Androgenetic Alopecia

- **OVERVIEW** 159
- **CHINESE MEDICAL ETIOLOGY AND PATHOMECHANISM** 161
- **CHINESE MEDICAL TREATMENT** 161
  - **Pattern Differentiation and Treatment** 162
  - **Additional Treatment Modalities** 167
    1. Chinese Patent Medicine 167
    2. Acupuncture and Moxibustion 169
    3. External Treatment 171
    4. Simple Prescriptions and Empirical Formulas 173
- **PROGNOSIS** 174
- **PREVENTIVE HEALTHCARE** 174
  - **Lifestyle Modification** 174
  - **Dietary Recommendation** 175
  - **Regulation of Emotional and Mental Health** 178
- **CLINICAL EXPERIENCE OF RENOWNED PHYSICIANS** 178
  - **Empirical Formulas** 178
    1. Yī Zhī Xǐ Fāng (溢脂洗方) (Zhu Ren-kang) 178
    2. Qū Shī Jiàn Fà Tāng (祛湿健发汤) (Zhao Bing-nan) 179
    3. Shēng Fà Tāng (生发汤) (Wang Jun-kang) 180
    4. Yǎng Xuè Rùn Zào Fāng (养血润燥方) (Li Jin-yong) 182
  - **Selected Case Studies** 182
    1. Case Studies of Zhang Zhi-li: Exuberant Dampness due to Spleen Deficiency, Wind Dryness due to Blood Deficiency 182
    2. Case Studies of Zhu Ren-kang: Heat in the Muscles with Wind Invasion, Impairing Yin and Exhausting Blood 185
    3. Case Studies of Xuan Guo-wei: Damp-Heat and Blood Heat ... 186
    4. Case Studies of Hu Guo-jun: Congealing Yin Cold 188
    5. Case Studies of Bai Ya-ping: Weak Nutritive Qi and Strong Defensive Qi ... 189
    6. Case Studies of Yu Wen-qiu: Yin Essence Deficiency, Spleen and Stomach Damp-heat 191

Discussions · · · · · · 192
1. ZHAO BING-NAN: TWO-PATTERN DIFFERENTIATION AND TREATMENT OF ANDROGENETIC ALOPECIA · · · · · · 192
2. CHEN DA-CHAN: CLINICAL EXPERIENCES OF ANDROGENETIC ALOPECIA · · · · · · 194
3. YU WEN-QIU: TREATMENT OF ANDROGENETIC ALOPECIA · · · · · · 198

PERSPECTIVES OF INTEGRATIVE MEDICINE · · · · · · 200
Challenges and Solutions · · · · · · 200
CHALLENGE #1: HOW TO CONTROL ALOPECIA · · · · · · 201
CHALLENGE #2: HOW TO DECREASE THE SEBUM SECRETION · · · · · · 201
CHALLENGE #3: HOW TO IMPROVE HAIR GROWTH · · · · · · 202

Insight from Empirical Wisdom · · · · · · 202
1. MODIFICATIONS ACCORDING TO CHANGES IN THE SYNDROME · · · · · · 203
2. INSIGHT FOR TREATMENT AND MEDICINAL APPLICATION · · · · · · 204
3. COMBINING INTERNAL AND EXTERNAL TREATMENT · · · · · · 205
4. ADHERENCE TO TREATMENT · · · · · · 206

Summary · · · · · · 206
SELECTED QUOTES FROM CLASSICAL TEXTS · · · · · · 206
MODERN RESEARCH · · · · · · 208
Clinical Research · · · · · · 208
1. PATTERN DIFFERENTIATION AND CORRESPONDING TREATMENT · · · · · · 208
2. SPECIFIC FORMULAS · · · · · · 214
3. ACUPUNCTURE AND MOXIBUSTION · · · · · · 218

Experimental Studies · · · · · · 220
1. RESEARCH ON THE EFFICACY OF SINGLE CHINESE MEDICINALS · · · · · · 220
2. RESEARCH ON THE EFFICACY OF HERBAL PRESCRIPTIONS · · · · · · 222
3. SYNDROME DIFFERENTIATION STUDIES · · · · · · 225

REFERENCES · · · · · · 225

OVERVIEW

　　Androgenetic alopecia is characterized by the slow development of hair loss, starting above both temples. It moves gradually to affect the forehead and/or vertex region, usually appearing after adolescence. Androgenetic alopecia is also known as seborrheic alopecia, male pattern alopecia, or disseminated alopecia. It can occur in both men and women, but is seen much more commonly in men. This type of alopecia is often accompanied with excessive sebaceous secretion, profuse seborrhea, excessive scales, dry hair, itchiness, and other symptoms. Because this disease is detrimental to the patients' self-image, most people seek medical treatment despite the financial cost.

　　The pathogenesis of androgenetic alopecia is quite complex. Modern medicine does not have a clear grasp of this disorder. It is thought that this type of genetic alopecia depends on androgens. There are many factors that play important roles with alopecia conditions, particularly related to androgen. These factors include androgens (testosterone, particularly an androgen called dihydrotestosterone), hair follicle monagastic androgen acceptor, enzyme activity (mainly 5α-reductase), and the genetic susceptibility of the alopecia scalp (target organ). Other factors that can lead to or worsen alopecia include emotions, diet, and infections. When young men between the ages of 20-30 have this type of alopecia, there is usually a family history present. Hair loss typically starts from the both sides of the forehead, progressing slowly towards the vertex. The hair is initially greasy or dry, and later becomes thinner and less in amount. New hair grows in thin and fine without much lustre. Some patients begin to display sudden hair loss at the vertex of the scalp initially. In these cases, it is often accompanied with excessive scales (dandruff), a grey desquamation in small pieces. These patients have no other symptoms except slight itching. Although the course of this disorder is slow, the rate of disease progression, affected areas, and severity varies from person to person. Symptoms can continue to linger for many years, or it can develop into alopecia senilis which can lead to permanent alopecia. This condition also occurs in females, but it is quite rare and also less severe. For women, the hair loss is more diffuse on the vertex, rarely appearing on the both sides of the forehead. It is also seldom that women develop permanent baldness.

There are no set standards of examination for the diagnosis of alopecia. The most common tests and examinations for alopecia include:

1) Tests for endocrine function
2) Tests for the microcirculation on the skin of the head
3) Hair trace element tests
4) Tests for tissue pathology, hormone levels, and enzyme activity

Both internal and external treatments are utilized for androgenetic alopecia. There are 2 kinds of internal treatments:

1) Androgen receptor inhibitors such as progesterone, aldactone, and tagamet
2) 5-alpha-reductase inhibitors such as finasteride

There are 5 kinds of external treatments:

1) 2%-4% progesterone tinctures
2) 1% minoxidil cream or solution
3) 1%-2% ciclosporin solution
4) 0.025% retinoic acid (tretinoin) alcohol solution
5) 0.05% dienestrol (hexadiene estrone) tincture

For patients with baldness rated higher than Hamilton 5, surgical intervention such as hair transplantation, scalp reduction, or scalp expansion may be required.

CHINESE MEDICAL ETIOLOGY AND PATHOMECHANISM

The Chinese medical perspective on androgenetic alopecia varies depending on its particular stage. In the early stages, the condition is associated with blood heat and wind dryness, or damp-heat in the spleen and stomach. In later stages, alopecia is generally associated with liver and kidney deficiency. When heat in the blood combines with pathogenic wind, it can also transform into dryness. Yin and blood also become exhausted, failing to rise upward to nourish the hair. This will manifest with dry hair, hair loss, thin yellow hair, desquamation (shedding of the skin), and itching.

The overconsumption of alcohol and fatty or spicy foods also leads to spleen deficiency with impairment of the spleen and stomach's function of transporting and transforming fluids. Congealed fluids will transform into heat, and damp-heat will rise to deteriorate the hair follicle. This pattern manifests with severe itching, sticky hair, and shedding.

If the patient's constitution is inherently deficient, and he is also affected overthinking and worrying, this will impair the liver and kidney. Essence and blood become deficient and cannot nourish the hair, thereby causing hair loss. Alopecia shows pathological changes on the hair, but the origin of the disease stems from the *zang fu* organs. Androgenetic alopecia is usually closely related to the liver, spleen and kidney.

CHINESE MEDICAL TREATMENT

Based on the presenting syndrome, treatment can include cooling blood and expelling wind, strengthening the spleen and eliminating dampness, or tonifying the liver and kidney. External and internal treatments are often combined, where acupuncture and herbal treatments are prescribed simultaneously.

Pattern Differentiation and Treatment

(1) Blood Heat and Wind Dryness

【Syndrome Characteristics】

Dry lusterless hair, hair shedding, white scales, sensation of heat on the head, scalp itchiness, dry mouth and throat, and yellow urine. The tongue is red with a slight yellow or dry coating, and the pulse is rapid.

【Treatment Principle】

Cool blood and clear heat, dispel wind and moisten dryness.

【Commonly Used Medicinals】

Shēng dì huáng (Radix Rehmanniae), *dān shēn* (Radix et Rhizoma Salviae Miltiorrhizae), and *dān pí* (Cortex Moutan) cool blood and clear heat. *Jīng jiè* (Herba Schizonepetae), *fáng fēng* (Radix Saposhnikoviae), *jí lí* (Fructus Tribuli), and *chán tuì* (Periostracum Cicadae) act to dispel wind.

【Representative Formula】

Modified *Liáng Xuè Xiāo Fēng Sǎn* (凉血消风散).

【Ingredients】

生地黄	shēng dì huáng	12g	Radix Rehmanniae
杭菊花	háng jú huā	12g	Flos Chrysanthemi
荆芥	jīng jiè	6g	Herba Schizonepetae
防风	fáng fēng	9g	Radix Saposhnikoviae
蝉蜕	chán tuì	6g	Periostracum Cicadae
刺蒺藜	jí lí	12g	Fructus Tribuli
苦参	kǔ shēn	6g	Radix Sophorae Flavescentis
白鲜皮	bái xiān pí	12g	Cortex Dictamni
当归	dāng guī	12g	Radix Angelicae Sinensis
甘草	gān cǎo	6g	Radix et Rhizoma Glycyrrhizae

Decoct in 500 ml of water until 100 ml remains. Take warm, twice a day.

【Formula Analysis】

Jú huā (Flos Chrysanthemi) is the chief herb that clears heat, dispels wind, and opens orifices. *Jīng jiè* (Herba Schizonepetae), *fáng fēng* (Radix Saposhnikoviae), *jí lí* (Fructus Tribuli), and *chán tuì* (Periostracum Cicadae) dispel wind, clear heat, relieve itching, and regrow hair. *Kǔ shēn* (Radix Sophorae Flavescentis) and *bái xiān pí* (Cortex Dictamni) clear heat and remove dampness. *Shēng dì huáng* (Radix Rehmanniae) clears heat and cools blood. *Dāng guī* (Radix Angelicae Sinensis) nourishes blood and moistens dryness. *Gān cǎo* (Radix et Rhizoma Glycyrrhizae) harmonizes all the herbs in the formula. All the herbs combined work together to cool blood, clear heat, dispel wind, moisten dryness, and regrow hair.

【Modifications】

➢ With exuberant heat in the blood level manifesting with five-center heat, and a red or crimson tongue, add *chì sháo* (Radix Paeoniae Rubra) 15g, *mǔ dān pí* (Cortex Moutan) 15g, and *zǐ cǎo* (Radix Arnebiae) 12g to clear heat and cool blood.

➢ With wind-heat manifesting with generalized fever, thirst, and redness on the scalp, add *jīn yín huā* (Flos Lonicerae Japonicae) 20g, and *lián qiào* (Fructus Forsythiae) 12g to course wind, clear heat, and resolve toxins.

➢ With dry hair, add *sāng shèn* (Fructus Mori) 15g, *tù sī zǐ* (Semen Cuscutae) 15g, and *hé shǒu wū* (Radix Polygoni Multiflori) 15g to tonify the liver and kidney, nourish blood, and moisten hair.

(2) Damp-heat Accumulation

【Syndrome Characteristics】

The patient usually reports the excessive consumption of greasy, sweet and rich foods. Manifestations include thin falling hair, excessive scales with scalp itchiness red scalp, dry mouth, bitter taste in the mouth, irritability, and a poor appetite. The tongue is red with a yellow greasy coating, and the pulse is wiry and slippery.

【Treatment Principle】

Clear heat, dispel dampness, and strengthen the spleen.

【Commonly Used Medicinals】

Fú líng (Poria), *zé xiè* (Rhizoma Alismatis) and *yì yǐ rén* (Semen Coicis) strengthen the spleen and dispel dampness. *Yīn chén* (Herba Artemisiae Scopariae), *bì xiè* (Rhizoma Dioscoreae Hypoglaucae), and *pú gōng yīng* (Herba Taraxaci) clear heat and drain dampness.

【Representative Formula】

Modified *Bì Xiè Shèn Shī Tāng* (萆薢渗湿汤)

【Ingredients】

萆薢	bì xiè	12g	Rhizoma Dioscoreae Hypoglaucae
茵陈蒿	yīn chén	15g	Herba Artemisiae Scopariae
白鲜皮	bái xiān pí	12g	Cortex Dictamni
炒白术	bái zhú	12g	Rhizoma Atractylodis Macrocephalae (dry-fried)
茯苓	fú líng	12g	Poria
泽泻	zé xiè	12g	Rhizoma Alismatis
炒薏苡仁	yì yǐ rén	15g	Semen Coicis (dry-fried)
生山楂	shān zhā	12g	Fructus Crataegi (raw)
赤石脂	chì shí zhī	9g	Halloysitum Rubrum
生地黄	shēng dì huáng	12g	Radix Rehmanniae
蒲公英	pú gōng yīng	30g	Herba Taraxaci
甘草	gān cǎo	6g	Radix et Rhizoma Glycyrrhizae

Decoct in 500 ml of water until 100 ml remains. Take warm, twice a day.

【Formula Analysis】

Bì xiè (Rhizoma Dioscoreae Hypoglaucae) is the chief herb that clears heat and drains dampness. *Yīn chén* (Herba Artemisiae Scopariae) and *bái xiān pí* (Cortex Dictamni) clear heat and dispel dampness. *Bái zhú* (dry-fried Rhizoma Atractylodis Macrocephalae), *fú líng* (Poria), *zé xiè* (Rhizoma Alismatis), and *yì yǐ rén* (dry-fried Semen Coicis) strengthen the spleen and eliminate dampness. *Shān zhā* (Fructus Crataegi) and *chì shí zhī* (Halloysitum Rubrum) eliminate dampness and fat. *Shēng dì huáng* (Radix Rehmanniae) and *pú gōng yīng* (Herba Taraxaci) clear heat and grow hair. *Gān cǎo* (Radix et Rhizoma Glycyrrhizae) clears heat, removes toxins, and harmonizes all the herbs in the formula. All the herbs work together to clear heat, dispel dampness, strengthen the spleen, and benefit the hair.

【Modifications】
> With greasy or oily hair, add *fú líng* (Poria) 15g, *mài yá* (Fructus Hordei Germinatus) 15g, and *bù zhā yè* (Microcoris Folium) 15g to eliminate dampness and fat.

> With profuse sweating on the scalp, add *wǔ wèi zǐ* (Fructus Schisandrae Chinensis) 12g and *sāng yè* (Folium Mori) 15g to disperse wind, clear heat, and astringe sweating.

(3) Liver and Kidney Deficiency
【Syndrome Characteristics】
This syndrome is most common among patients with a weak constitution, or those with stressful professional jobs that require excessive thinking. Manifestations include hair loss, balding areas, or sparse hair. Other symptoms include dizziness, insomnia, poor memory, soreness and weakness of the lower back and knees, and profuse or frequent urination in the night. The tongue is light red with scant coating, and the pulse is thready and deep.

With yin deficiency, manifestations include a bitter taste in the mouth, five-center heat, profuse dreaming, and nocturnal emission. The tongue is red with a scant coating, and the pulse is rapid and thready.

【Treatment Principle】
Tonify the liver and kidney to nourish and regrow hair.

【Commonly Used Medicinals】
To tonify the liver and kidney, *zhì hé shǒu wū* (Radix Polygoni

Multiflori Praeparata cum Succo Glycines Sotae), *tù sī zǐ* (Semen Cuscutae), *shān zhū yú* (Fructus Corni), *gǒu qǐ zǐ* (Fructus Lycii), *nǚ zhēn zǐ* (Fructus Ligustri Lucidi), *hàn lián cǎo* (Herba Ecliptae), and *huáng jīng* (Rhizoma Polygonati) can be selected.

【Representative Formula】

Modified *Qī Bǎo Měi Rán Dān* (七宝美髯丹)

【Ingredients】

制何首乌	zhì hé shǒu wū	15g	Radix Polygoni Multiflori Praeparata cum Succo Glycines Sotae
枸杞子	gǒu qǐ zǐ	9g	Fructus Lycii
菟丝子	tù sī zǐ	18g	Semen Cuscutae
黄精	huáng jīng	12g	Rhizoma Polygonati
山茱萸	shān zhū yú	9g	Fructus Corni
黄芪	huáng qí	18g	Radix Astragali
党参	dǎng shēn	12g	Radix Codonopsis
白术	bái zhú	12g	Rhizoma Atractylodis Macrocephalae
女贞子	nǚ zhēn zǐ	18g	Fructus Ligustri Lucidi
旱莲草	hàn lián cǎo	18g	Herba Ecliptae
当归	dāng guī	15g	Radix Angelicae Sinensis
炙甘草	zhì gān cǎo	6g	Radix et Rhizoma Glycyrrhizae Praeparata cum Melle

Decoct in 500 ml of water until 100 ml remains. Take warm, twice a day.

【Formula Analysis】

Zhì hé shǒu wū (Radix Polygoni Multiflori Praeparata cum Succo Glycines Sotae) is the chief herb that tonifies the liver and kidney, benefits essence and blood, darkens the hair color, and strengthens sinews and bones. *Tù sī zǐ* (Semen Cuscutae), *shān zhū yú* (Fructus Corni), *gǒu qǐ zǐ* (Fructus Lycii), and *huáng jīng* (Rhizoma Polygonati) are deputy herbs that tonify the kidney and benefit essence, nourish liver and blood, and tonify congenital deficiencies. The assistant herbs are *huáng qí*

(Radix Astragali), *dǎng shēn* (Radix Codonopsis) and *bái zhú* (Rhizoma Atractylodis Macrocephalae) which benefit qi and tonify the spleen. The assistant herbs include *nǚ zhēn zǐ* (Fructus Ligustri Lucidi) and *hàn lián cǎo* (Herba Ecliptae) to tonify yin to regrow hair, and *dāng guī* (Radix Angelicae Sinensis) invigorates and nourishes blood to regrow hair. *Zhì gān cǎo* (Radix et Rhizoma Glycyrrhizae Praeparata cum Melle) tonifies earth and harmonizes all the other herbs in the formula. All the herbs work together to tonify yin and essence, and nourish blood to regrow hair.

【Modifications】

➤ With soreness and weakness of the back and knees, dizziness, and tinnitus, add *sāng jì shēng* (Herba Taxilli) 15g, and *xù duàn* (Radix Dipsaci) 12g to tonify kidney and invigorate yang.

➤ With yin deficiency, select *Liù Wèi Dì Huáng Wán* (六味地黄丸) plus *nǚ zhēn zǐ* (Fructus Ligustri Lucidi) 18g, and *hàn lián cǎo* (Herba Ecliptae) 18g to tonify the liver and kidney, nourish yin, and clear heat. *Nǚ zhēn zǐ* (Fructus Ligustri Lucidi) and *hàn lián cǎo* (Herba Ecliptae) act to strengthen the kidney and nourish yin to nourish and grow hair.

Additional Treatment Modalities

1. Chinese Patent Medicine

(1) *Yǎng Xuè Shēng Fà Jiāo Náng* (养血生发胶囊)

Take 4 capsules each time, 3 times a day with warm water. Nourishes blood, tonifies the kidney, dispels wind, and regrows hair. Indicated for alopecia due to essence and blood deficiency with wind.

(2) *Hé Shǒu Wū Piàn* (何首乌片)

Take 5 pills each time, 3 times a day with warm water. Tonifies the liver and kidney, and darkens hair color. Indicated for alopecia due to liver and kidney deficiency.

(3) *Liù Wèi Dì Huáng Wán* (六味地黄丸)

Take 6g each time, 3 times a day with warm water. Tonifies the liver and kidney. Indicated for alopecia due to liver and kidney deficiency.

(4) *Lóng Dǎn Xiè Gān Wán* (龙胆泻肝丸)

Take 6g, 2-3 times a day with warm water. Clears fire from the liver and gall bladder, and clears damp-heat from the triple burner. Indicated for excessive heat in liver and gall bladder.

(5) *Jiàn Pí Wán* (健脾丸)

Take 6g one time, 2-3 times a day, take with warm water. Strengthens the spleen and eliminates dampness. Indicated for spleen deficiency with excessive dampness.

(6) *Qū Zhī Shēng Fà Wán* (祛脂生发丸)

One pill each time, 2 times a day with warm water. Indicated for damp-heat in the spleen and stomach.

(7) *Èr Zhì Wán* (二至丸)

Take 6g each time, 2 times a day with warm water. Tonifies the liver and kidney, and darkens the hair and beard. Indicated for liver and kidney deficiency.

(8) *Líng Dān Piàn* (灵丹片)

Take 4 pills each time, 3 times a day with warm water. Indicated to prevent alopecia and benefit hair growth.

(9) *Fú Sāng Piàn* (扶桑片)

Take 6g each time, 2-3 times a day with warm water. It darkens the hair and improves the appearance. Indicated for exuberant wind and damp obstruction.

2. Acupuncture and Moxibustion

(1) Acupuncture

【Point Combination】

DU 20	bǎi huì	百会
EX-HN1	sì shén cōng	四神聪
ST 8 (bilaterally)	tóu wéi	头维（双）
(the midpoints of GB 20 and DU 16, bilaterally)	shēng fà xuè	生发穴
SJ 17	yì fēng	翳风

【Manipulation】

Use supplementation or drainage techniques based on the individual constitution. Retain all needles for 20 minutes; electro-stimulation is applicable. Treatment are given daily, or once every other day. Ten days constitute one course of treatment.

(2) Ear Acupuncture

【Point Combination】

lung	CO14	fèi	肺
kidney	CO10	shèn	肾
sympathetic	AH6a	jiāo gǎn	交感

【Manipulation】

Needle once every other day, or use ear seeds.

(3) 3-needle Scalp Acupuncture

【Point Combination】

Select these two points as basic points:

fáng lǎo（防老）	one *cun* posterior to DU 20 (*bǎi huì*)
jiàn nǎo xuè（健脑穴）	0.5 *cun* below GB 20 (*fēng chí*)

【Point Modifications】

With excessive sebum secretion, add DU 23 (*shàng xīng*).

With an itchy scalp, add DU 14 (*dà zhuī*).

【Manipulation】

When needling the *fáng lǎo* (防老) point, be sure the needle is directed towards the anterior hairline and angled subcutaneously 0.1 *cun* beneath the scalp. Treat daily or every other day for 15-30 minutes. Ten treatments constitute one course of treatment.

(4) Plum-blossom Needle and TDP Therapeutic Apparatus

【Point Combination】

alopecia area		头部脱发区
DU 20	*bǎi huì*	百会
GB 20	*fēng chí*	风池

【Manipulation】

First, use 75% alcohol to clean the affected area. Then apply gentle plum-blossom needling uniformly on the affected areas, DU 20, and GB 20. It is not advisable to bleed these areas. Depending on the skin condition, tap these areas for 3-5 min. Then apply a TDP lamp at 20-30 cm, or whatever distance is comfortable for the patient. Treat for 15-20 minutes, twice per week.

【Function】

Free the channels and collaterals, move qi and activate blood, disperse stasis, and nourish qi, blood and fluids to promote hair.

(5) Scalp Tapping Therapy

【Manipulation】

Using a plum blossom needle, tap along the following areas. First, taking the governing vessel as the midline, from the top of the ears, draw 2 parallel lines. Second, draw a perpendicular line between the top of ear and the governing vessel. At this point, the head is divided into four parts. They are identified as the governing vessel line, left line, right line, left base line, and right base line. Tap the scalp on these lines; 3 times a day for 15 consecutive days; as one course of treatment. This therapy has shown good clinical effects on mild to moderate cases.

3. External Treatment

(1) External Wash

A. Select the formula for external washing based on the dryness or greasiness of the hair.

➤ For damp-heat manifesting with greasy hair, select *Tòu Gǔ Cǎo Fāng* (透骨草方) or *Zhī Yì Xǐ Fāng* (脂溢洗方).

a. *Tòu Gǔ Cǎo Fāng* (透骨草方):

透骨草	tòu gǔ cǎo	20g	Caulis Impatientis
侧柏叶	cè bǎi yè	20g	Cacumen Platycladi
皂角刺	zào jiǎo cì	60g	Spina Gleditsiae
白矾	bái fán	10g	Alumen

Decoct with water and wash over the affected areas.

b. *Zhī Yì Xǐ Fāng* (脂溢洗方):

苍耳子	cāng ěr zǐ	30g	Fructus Xanthii
王不留行	wáng bù liú xíng	30g	Semen Vaccariae
苦参	kǔ shēn	15g	Radix Sophorae Flavescentis
白矾	bái fán	9g	Alumen

Decoct with water and wash over the affected areas.

➤ For excessive wind dryness manifesting with dry hair, select *Sāng Bái Pí Xǐ Fāng* (桑白皮洗方):

桑白皮	sāng bái pí	30g	Cortex Mori
五倍子	wǔ bèi zǐ	15g	Galla Chinensis
青葙子	qīng xiāng zǐ	60g	Semen Celosiae

Decoct with water and wash over the affected areas.

B. External wash for seborrheic dermatitis:

| 野菊花 | yě jú huā | 20g | Flos Chrysanthemi Indici |

| 白芷 | bái zhǐ | 15g | Radix Angelicae Dahuricae |
| 薄荷 | bò hé | 15g | Herba Menthae (decoct later) |

Apply once every 3-5 days.

C. External wash to relieve itchy scalp and dandruff:

苍耳子	cāng ěr zǐ	30g	Fructus Xanthii
王不留行	wáng bù liú xíng	30g	Semen Vaccariae
苦参	kǔ shēn	15g	Radix Sophorae Flavescentis
明矾	bái fán	9g	Alumen

Apply once every three days.

(2) External Liniment

A. *Pí Zhī Cā Jì* (皮脂擦剂):

硫黄	liú huáng	10g	Sulfur
枯矾	kū fán	2g	Alumen dehydratum
轻粉	qīng fěn	2g	Calomelas

Mix the above medicinals with 10% *dà huáng* (Radix et Rhizoma Rhei) water. Apply to the scalp twice a day.

B. *Tuō Fà Zài Shēng Jì* (脱发再生剂):

鲜侧柏叶	cè bǎi yè	40g	Cacumen Platycladi (fresh)
何首乌	hé shǒu wū	10g	Radix Polygoni Multiflori
白鲜皮	bái xiān pí	10g	Cortex Dictamni
毛姜	máo jiāng	10g	Rhizoma Drynariae

Soak the above herbs in 200 ml of 75% alcohol for 2 weeks. Apply the liquid to the affected areas.

C. *Bīng Fà Shēng Zhǎng Fāng* (鬓发生长方): mash equal amounts of *sāng yè* (Folium Mori) and *má yè* (Cannabis Folium). Soak in 75% alcohol with a 30% proportion of herbs to alcohol. Soak for one week. Apply the liquid to the affected areas and massage into the scalp for 3 minutes, twice a day.

D. Grind the peels of *shēng jiāng* (Rhizoma Zingiberis Recens) 50g and *rén shēn* (Radix Ginseng) 50g into powder. Take a separate piece of fresh *shēng jiāng*; dip into the powder, and rub onto the affected areas.

E. *Shēng Fà Dīng* (生发酊)

川花椒	huā jiāo	20g	Pericarpium Zanthoxyli
侧柏叶	cè bǎi yè	20g	Cacumen Platycladi
老生姜	shēng jiāng	20g	Rhizoma Zingiberis Recens
红花	hóng huā	20g	Flos Carthami

Soak in 75% alcohol for 20 days. Apply the tincture to the affected area 1-2 times a day.

F. *Shēng Fà Jiǔ* (生发酒)

| 斑蝥 | bān máo | 2 pieces | Mylabris |
| 百部 | bǎi bù | 20g | Radix Stemonae |

Soak in 100 ml of 75% alcohol for 7 days. Apply the liquid to the affected local areas twice a day.

G. *Xiāng Jú Jiǔ* (香菊酒)

零陵香	líng líng xiāng	20g	fenugreek lysimachia
香白芷	xiāng bái zhǐ	20g	Radix Angelicae Dahuricae
野菊花	yě jú huā	15g	Flos Chrysanthemi Indici
甘松	gān sōng	10g	Radix et Rhizoma Nardostachyos
防风	fáng fēng	10g	Radix Saposhnikoviae

Soak in 400 ml of 60% alcohol for 3 days. Apply the liquid to the affected areas twice a day.

H. *Wú Gōng* Oil (蜈蚣油) Apply the oil to the scalp 1-2 times a day. Indicated for long-term or serious cases of thinning hair; or alopecia at an early age.

4. Simple Prescriptions and Empirical Formulas

(1) Decoct *zhī má gěng* (sesame stem) 100g and *qīng míng liǔ* (the

tender willow leaf picked during Qing Ming festival) 100g with water. Wash the hair and massage into the scalp. Use for 1-2 months.

(2) *Bīng Fà Duò Luò Lìng Shēng Zhǎng Fāng* (鬓发堕落令生长方): *sāng yè* (Folium Mori) 500g and *má yè* (Cannabis Folium) 500g. Grind the herbs into powder and soak in 75% alcohol with a 30% proportion of herbs to alcohol. Soak for one week. Apply the liquid to the affected areas and massage for 3 minutes. Twice a day for 3 months constitutes one course of treatment. Indicated for dry or greasy type androgenetic alopecia.

(3) Decoct *dà huáng* (Radix et Rhizoma Rhei) 10g, *huáng qín* (Radix Scutellariae) 15g, and *huáng lián* (Rhizoma Coptidis) 15g. Indicated for androgenetic alopecia due to damp-heat.

(4) Grind 120g raw *dài zhě shí* (Haematitum) into powder. Apply 3g onto the affected areas, twice a day.

PROGNOSIS

Androgenetic alopecia has a slow progression. Clinical treatment mainly focuses on slowing the progression, and addressing the condition of the oily, itchy scalp. Clinical efficacy is measured by the degree of hair loss and decrease of oily hair, scalp itching, and desquamation. Chinese medicine is certainly beneficial for delaying the progression of alopecia conditions. Clinical experience shows high efficacy for alopecia in the early stages and moderate effectiveness on alopecia in the middle stages. For late-stage alopecia, hair transplantation seems to be the most successful method for restoring the desired appearance.

PREVENTIVE HEALTHCARE

Lifestyle Modification

(1) Proper cleaning of the hair and scalp: It is important to regularly wash the skin to remove sebum, sweat or other kinds of toxins that excrete from the skin. Assure your patients that healthy hair will not fall out with regular hair-washing. Washing of the hair 1-2 times a week is sufficient in the colder season; more often in the summer. It is best to use water with the least amount of mineral content, because soft water is not as irritating to the scalp. The best water temperature for hair washing is close to body temperature. Oily hair should be cleaned with a shampoo that contains sulfur or boric acid, because these two elements can remove oils. Dry hair is brittle and easy to break, so for this type of hair, it is best to avoid alkaline-based shampoos.

(2) Hair salon products: If the hair is already oily, the use of cream or oil-based hair products can worsen alopecia conditions. However, these products are appropriate for those with dry hair.

(3) Avoid strong physical stimulation: It is best to avoid stimulation of the hair follicles by scratching, using a hard comb, or wearing hats for long periods of time. Moderate exposure to the sun and scalp massages are recommended. However, hats are recommended for those individuals who work outdoors to prevent overexposure to wind, dryness, and sun.

Dietary Recommendation

Foods with high protein and vitamins such as milk, egg, meat, fish, beans, seafood, fresh vegetables, and fruits are recommended. For patients with oily secretions, they should eat more fresh foods, fibers and grains. Eating *shān zhā* (Fructus Crataegi) or strawberries can also help control greasy hair. It is generally best to limit greasy and fatty foods, animal fats and organs, carbohydrates, strong teas, spicy foods, and condiments such as pepper and garlic.

Vitamin A plays an important role in maintaining the structure, function, and growth of the epithelial tissue. Foods high in vitamin A include carrots, spinach, cabbage, chives, celery, and apricots.

Vitamin B6 regulates the synthesis of fatty acids and fats, prevents sebum secretion, and helps the hair to grow. Foods high in Vitamin B6 include potatoes, green beans, herring, oranges, and sesame.

Seaweed is rich in iodine and also good for healthy hair. Cooking it with oil can facilitate the absorption of iodine.

The following herbs may be added to the daily diet:

➤ Herbs that improve hair growth: *sāng shèn* (Fructus Mori), *sāng jì shēng* (Herba Taxilli), *hàn lián cǎo* (Herba Ecliptae), *dōng guā zǐ* (Semen Benincasae), *xīn yí huā* (Flos Magnoliae), and *fú píng* (Herba Spirodelae).

➤ Herbs that nourish hair: *gān dì huáng* (Radix Rehmanniae), *bǎi zǐ rén* (Semen Platycladi), *nǚ zhēn zǐ* (Fructus Ligustri Lucidi), *qín jiāo* (Radix Gentianae Macrophyllae), *shā shēn* (Radix Glehniae/Adenophorae), *yù zhú* (Rhizoma Polygonati Odorati), *bái zhú* (Rhizoma Atractylodis Macrocephalae), *bái zhǐ* (Radix Angelicae Dahuricae), *guā lóu* (Fructus Trichosanthis), and *gǎo běn* (Rhizoma et Radix Ligustici).

➤ Herbs that darken the hair: *hé shǒu wū* (Radix Polygoni Multiflori), *fù pén zǐ* (Fructus Rubi), *tiān dōng* (Radix Asparagi), *mài dōng* (Radix Ophiopogonis), *nǚ zhēn zǐ* (Fructus Ligustri Lucidi), *huáng jīng* (Rhizoma Polygonati), *shú dì huáng* (Radix Rehmanniae Praeparata), and *hú táo* (Semen Juglandis).

(1) Pig Kidney and Walnut (猪肾核桃)

猪肾	zhū shèn	1 pair	pig kidneys
杜仲	dù zhòng	30g	Cortex Eucommiae
沙苑蒺藜	shā yuàn jí lí	15g	Semen Astragali Complanati
核桃仁	hé táo rén	30g	Semen Juglandis

Cook with high heat for 30 minutes, and then lower the flame until it is fully cooked. Drink the broth and eat the kidneys and walnuts. Take once a day for 7-10 consecutive days. This recipe is indicated for alopecia due to kidney yin deficiency. Symptoms and signs include dizziness, forgetfulness, tinnitus, deafness, five-center heat, insomnia, profuse dreaming, scant tongue coating, and a thready and rapid pulse.

(2) Black Bean and Pear Soup (黑豆雪梨汤)

Add the following foods to a pot of water: black beans 30g, and 1 or 2 sliced pears. Bring to a boil and then simmer over a low flame until fully cooked. Drink the broth, and eat the pears. Take twice a day for 15-17 consecutive days.

This recipe is indicated for alopecia due to lung yin deficiency. Symptoms and signs include thinning hair, pale complexion, fatigue, and the tendency to catch colds easily.

(3) *Băi Hé Xìng Rén Zhōu* (百合杏仁粥)

百合	băi hé	50g	Bulbus Lilii
杏仁	xìng rén	10g	Armeniacae Semen Amarum
粳米	jīng mǐ	50g	Oryza sativa L.

Cook the *jīng mǐ* (Oryza sativa L.) into porridge, then add *xìng rén* (Armeniacae Semen Amarum) and *băi hé* (Bulbus Lilii) and cook until soft. Eat once a day for 15-30 consecutive days.

This recipe is indicated for alopecia due to lung qi deficiency. Symptoms and signs include hair that easy falls out, asthma, cough, fatigue, clear phlegm, a low weak voice, and a light red tongue with a thin white coating.

(4) *Guì Yuán Lián Zǐ Zhōu* (桂圆莲子粥)

龙眼肉	lóng yăn ròu	10g	Arillus Longan
莲子	lián zǐ	15g	Semen Nelumbinis
大枣	dà zăo	10 pieces	Fructus Jujubae
粳米	jīng mǐ	50g	Oryza sativa L.

Cook all ingredients into porridge. Eat twice a day for 15-30 consecutive days.

This recipe is indicated for alopecia due to qi and blood deficiency.

Symptoms and signs include dry yellowish hair that falls out easily, palpitations, shortness of breath, spontaneous sweating, night sweating, pale tongue, scant tongue coating, and a thready, weak pulse.

(5) *Wū Dòu Táng Shī Bǎo* (乌豆塘虱煲)

| 乌豆 | wū dòu | 60g | Semen Sojae Nigrum |
| 塘虱 | táng shī | 2 pieces | catfish |

Clean one catfish, removing the head, and boil with black beans until well cooked. Add salt or oil to taste.

Indicated for all types kinds of alopecia.

Regulation of Emotional and Mental Health

Regulating the emotions and mind is also important in the treatment of alopecia. Patients should avoid emotional stress and excessive mental work if possible. It is important to maintain a healthy lifestyle with sufficient time for relaxation. Also beneficial is to cultivate a sense of overall contentment, to be open-minded, to have sufficient sleep, and to do regular exercise. Since results may not suddenly emerge, patients should be encouraged to remain persistent, and continue with treatment.

CLINICAL EXPERIENCE OF RENOWNED PHYSICIANS

Empirical Formulas

1. *Yì Zhī Xǐ Fāng* (溢脂洗方) (Zhu Ren-kang)

【Ingredients】

苍耳子	cāng ěr zǐ	30g	Fructus Xanthii
王不留行	wáng bù liú xíng	30g	Semen Vaccariae
苦参	kǔ shēn	15g	Radix Sophorae Flavescentis
明矾	míng fán	9g	Alumen

Decoct with water as an external wash. Apply once every 4 days. This wash acts to relieve itching and clean dandruff.

(Guang An Men Hospital of China Academy of Chinese Medical Sciences. *Clinical Experience Recordings of Zhu Ren-kang* (朱仁康临床经验集). Beijing: The People's Medical Publishing House, 1979, 290)

2. Qū Shī Jiàn Fà Tāng (祛湿健发汤) (Zhao Bing-nan)

【Ingredients】

炒白术	bái zhú	15g	Rhizoma Atractylodis Macrocephalae (dry-fried)
泽泻	zé xiè	10g	Rhizoma Alismatis
猪苓	zhū líng	15g	Polyporus
萆薢	bì xiè	15g	Rhizoma Dioscoreae Hypoglaucae
车前子	chē qián zǐ	10g	Semen Plantaginis
首乌藤	shǒu wū téng	15g	Caulis Polygoni Multiflori
川芎	chuān xiōng	10g	Rhizoma Chuanxiong
赤石脂	chì shí zhī	12g	Halloysitum Rubrum

Decoct in 500 ml of water until 100 ml remains. Take warm, twice a day.

【Indications】

Alopecia due to damp-heat, mainly manifesting with oily hair, or excessive dandruff and itching.

【Formula Analysis】

Bái zhú (dry-fried Rhizoma Atractylodis Macrocephalae), *zé xiè* (Rhizoma Alismatis), *zhū líng* (Polyporus), *bì xiè* (Rhizoma Dioscoreae Hypoglaucae), and *chē qián zǐ* (Semen Plantaginis) can strengthen the spleen and dispel dampness without impairing yin. *Chē qián zǐ* (Semen Plantaginis) drains damp, but also nourishes yin. *Shǒu wū téng* (Caulis Polygoni Multiflori) tonifies the kidney and nourishes blood to regrow hair. *Chuān xiōng* (Rhizoma Chuanxiong) moves blood and guides the medicinals upwards. *Chì shí zhī* (Halloysitum Rubrum) astringes to reduce oil secretions. All the medicinals work together to drain dampness, guide yin and blood upward, and strengthen both skin and the hair. This formula effectively treats both branch and root.

(Qin Han-kun. Syndromes and Treatment of Alopecia (脱发证治). *Journal of Traditional Chinese Medicine* (中医杂志), 1986,(12):10)

3. Shēng Fà Tāng (生发汤) (Wang Jun-kang)

【Ingredients】

何首乌（炙）	hé shǒu wū	10g	Radix Polygoni Multiflori (liquid-fried)
熟地黄	shú dì huáng	15g	Radix Rehmanniae Praeparata
当归	dāng guī	15g	Radix Angelicae Sinensis
生黄芪	shēng huáng qí	30g	Radix Astragali (raw)
枸杞子	gǒu qǐ zǐ	10g	Fructus Lycii
桑椹子	sāng shèn zǐ	10g	Fructus Mori
白鲜皮	bái xiān pí	10g	Cortex Dictamni
生地黄	shēng dì huáng	15g	Radix Rehmanniae
苦参	kǔ shēn	10g	Radix Sophorae Flavescentis
路路通	lù lù tōng	10g	Fructus Liquidambaris
板蓝根	bǎn lán gēn	10g	Radix Isatidis
桂枝尖	guì zhī	10g	Ramulus Cinnamomi

Decoct in 500 ml of water until 100 ml remains. Take warm, twice a day.

【Formula Analysis】

Hé shǒu wū (liquid-fried Radix Polygoni Multiflori) nourishes yin and blood, secures the kidney qi, and darkens the hair. *Shú dì huáng* (Radix Rehmanniae Praeparata) and *dāng guī* (Radix Angelicae Sinensis) nourish blood. *Huáng qí* (Radix Astragali) tonifies qi and strengthens immune function. *Gǒu qǐ zǐ* (Fructus Lycii) and *sāng shèn* (Fructus Mori) enrich the kidney and nourish yin. *Bái xiān pí* (Cortex Dictamni) dispels wind and relieves itching. *Shēng dì huáng* (Radix Rehmanniae), *kǔ shēn* (Radix Sophorae Flavescentis), and *bǎn lán gēn* (Radix Isatidis) cool blood and resolve toxins. *Lù lù tōng* (Fructus Liquidambaris) moves blood and frees the channels and collaterals. Modern research shows that *guì zhī* (Ramulus Cinnamomi) can dilate capillaries, regulate blood circulation, and move blood to the superficial layers of the skin. The kidney dominates hair, and hair is the extension of the blood. Hair needs blood to be sufficiently nourished. The herbs in the formula that nourish blood include *shú dì huáng* (Radix Rehmanniae Praeparata), *dāng guī* (Radix Angelicae Sinensis), and *hé shǒu wū* (liquid-fried Radix Polygoni Multiflori). These are used in large dosages to strongly tonify blood.

【Modifications】

➢ With spleen deficiency leading to damp encumbrance, add *fú líng* (Poria) 10g.

➢ With kidney deficiency, add *shān zhū yú* (Fructus Corni) 10g, *shān yào* (Rhizoma Dioscoreae) 10g, and *mǔ dān pí* (Cortex Moutan) 10g.

➢ With liver and kidney deficiency, add *nǚ zhēn zǐ* (Fructus Ligustri Lucidi) 10g, *hàn lián cǎo* (Herba Ecliptae) 10g, and *jí lí* (Fructus Tribuli) 10g.

➢ With yin and yang deficiency, add *Jīn Guì Shèn Qì Wán* (金匮肾气丸).

➢ With heart and spleen deficiency, add *Guī Pí Tāng* (归脾汤).

➢ With qi and blood deficiency, add *Bā Zhēn Tāng* (八珍汤).

➢ With liver constraint and blood deficiency, add *Xiāo Yáo Sǎn* (逍遥散).

➢ With blood heat engendering wind, add *Wū Fà Wán*, *dān shēn* (Radix et Rhizoma Salviae Miltiorrhizae) 10g, *bái sháo* (Radix Paeoniae Alba) 10g, and *jīng jiè* (Herba Schizonepetae) 10g. In addition, *Chú Zhī Líng* (除脂灵) may be selected for external application:

斑蝥	bān máo	2 pieces	Mylabris
狼毒	láng dú	10g	Radix Euphorbiae Fischerianae
川草乌	cǎo wū	10g	Radix Aconiti Kusnezoffii
麻黄	má huáng	10g	Herba Ephedrae
百部	bǎi bù	10g	Radix Stemonae

Soak all medicinals in 1000 ml of 75% alcohol for 1 week; apply the liquid externally.

(Zhang Jun-ting. Editor-in-chief. *Modern Chinese Medicine Doctors' Empirical Formulas* (当代中医师灵验奇方真传). Beijing: Chinese Medical Science and Technology Publishing House, 1994, 1144)

4. Yǎng Xuè Rùn Zào Fāng (养血润燥方) (Li Jin-yong)

【Ingredients】

何首乌	hé shǒu wū	20g	Radix Polygoni Multiflori
生地黄	shēng dì huáng	20g	Radix Rehmanniae
当归	dāng guī	10g	Radix Angelicae Sinensis
柏子仁	bǎi zǐ rén	10g	Semen Platycladi
蝉蜕	chán tuì	10g	Periostracum Cicadae
防风	fáng fēng	10g	Radix Saposhnikoviae
茯苓	fú líng	10g	Poria
旱莲草	hàn lián cǎo	15g	Herba Ecliptae
侧柏叶	cè bǎi yè	30g	Cacumen Platycladi

Decoct in 500 ml of water until 100 ml remains. Take warm, twice a day.

【Indications】

Blood dryness with wind; manifesting with hair falling out, baldness, excessive dandruff, and itching.

(Li Jin-yong. *Clinical Experience of Li Jin-yong* (李今庸临床经验辑要). Beijing: Chinese Medical Science and Technology Publishing House, 1998, 339)

Selected Case Studies

1. Case Studies of Zhang Zhi-li: Exuberant Dampness Due to Spleen Deficiency, Wind Dryness Due to Blood Deficiency

Ms. Liu, 49 years old.

【Initial Visit】

November 29th, 1987. The patient complained of excessive dandruff and itchiness of the scalp for about ten years. She had to wash her hair almost daily, otherwise her scalp would feel very itchy. In recent years, she displayed red macules, oily dandruff and itchiness on the nasolabial groove and around the supraorbital ridge. There was obvious hair loss at the top of her head.

Examination: thinning hair on the crown of the head with scales and dandruff. Some parts of scalp showed erythema with blood scabbed papules. The skin of the alae nasi, the nasolabial groove, and supraorbital ridge were rough with scales. The facial pores were large and oily. Pale tongue, white tongue coating, and a wiry and slippery pulse.

【Pattern Differentiation】

Exuberant dampness due to spleen deficiency, wind dryness due to blood deficiency, and hair deprived of nourishment.

【Treatment Principle】

Strengthen the spleen, eliminate dampness, nourish blood and moisten skin, regrow and strengthen hair.

【Prescription】

白术	bái zhú	10g	Rhizoma Atractylodis Macrocephalae
泽泻	zé xiè	10g	Rhizoma Alismatis
川芎	chuān xiōng	10g	Rhizoma Chuanxiong
牡丹皮	mǔ dān pí	10g	Cortex Moutan
当归	dāng guī	10g	Radix Angelicae Sinensis
赤芍	chì sháo	10g	Radix Paeoniae Rubra
白芍	bái sháo	10g	Radix Paeoniae Alba
何首乌	hé shǒu wū	10g	Radix Polygoni Multiflori
黑芝麻	hēi zhī ma	10g	Semen Sesami Nigrum
黑桑椹	sāng shèn	10g	Fructus Mori
天麻	tiān má	10g	Rhizoma Gastrodiae
薏苡仁	yì yǐ rén	30g	Semen Coicis
车前子	chē qián zǐ	15g	Semen Plantaginis
生地黄	shēng dì huáng	15g	Radix Rehmanniae
女贞子	nǚ zhēn zǐ	15g	Fructus Ligustri Lucidi
菟丝子	tù sī zǐ	15g	Semen Cuscutae

External Use: *Lù Liǔ* Tincture (氯柳酊) and *Shēng Fà Jiàn Fà* Tincture (生发健发酊) were used as alternating external washes. Sulfur Wash Preparation was selected for facial washing.

【Second Visit】

After 14 doses, the symptoms of itching, scales, oily hair and falling hair had all improved. After the second course of 14 doses, scalp itching was almost eliminated, and her hair stopped falling out.

To consolidate the therapeutic effects, the prescription was changed to Chinese patent medicines: *Chú Shī Wán* (除湿丸) 6g, twice a day and *Yǎng Xuè Shēng Fà Jiāo Náng* (养血生发胶囊) 3 pills, 3 times a day. The patient was also instructed to wash her hair less often.

Comments:

This patient had suffered from her condition for long time. Her yin and blood were exhausted, which led to blood deficiency and wind-dryness. Therefore, a prescription was chosen to strengthen the spleen and eliminate dampness, nourish blood and moisten dryness. In the formula, *bái zhú* (Rhizoma Atractylodis Macrocephalae), *yì yǐ rén* (Semen Coicis), *zé xiè* (Rhizoma Alismatis), and *chē qián zǐ* (Semen Coicis) were selected to tonify the spleen and eliminate dampness. *Dāng guī* (Radix Angelicae Sinensis), *chuān xiōng* (Rhizoma Chuanxiong), *shēng dì huáng* (Radix Rehmanniae), and *bái sháo* (Radix Paeoniae Alba) act to nourish the blood and moisten skin. *Nǚ zhēn zǐ* (Fructus Ligustri Lucidi), *tù sī zǐ* (Semen Cuscutae), *sāng shèn* (Fructus Mori), and *hēi zhī ma* (Semen Sesami Nigrum) were selected to nourish the kidney and enrich yin. *Tiān má* (Rhizoma Gastrodiae) and *chuān xiōng* (Rhizoma Chuanxiong) act to dispel wind and invigorate the blood.

(An Jia-feng Zhang Bi. Editors-in-chief. *Selected Case Studies of Zhang Zhi-li Treating Dermatological Diseases* (张志礼皮肤病医案选萃). Beijing: People's Medical Publishing House, 1994, 221)

2. Case Studies of Zhu Ren-kang: Heat in the Muscles with Wind Invasion, Impairing Yin and Exhausting Blood

Mr. Mao, 32 years old.

【Initial Visit】

The patient reported frequently washing his hair with cold water, which allowed a vulnerability for wind to easily invade. During the last year, he had begun to feel itchiness on his scalp. After scratching, scales and scabbing appeared. His forehead, ears, and face also began to display scales and scabbing.

Examination: red flushed patches and fine scales on the ears, neck, face, with larger patches on the scalp. Red tongue, scant coating, and a wiry slippery pulse.

【Pattern Differentiation】

Heat in muscles with wind invasion; leading to dryness impairing yin and exhausting blood.

【Treatment Principle】

Nourish yin and clear heat, moisten dryness, and relieve itching.

【Prescription】

生地黄	shēng dì huáng	30g	Radix Rehmanniae
玄参	xuán shēn	9g	Radix Scrophulariae
泽泻	zé xiè	9g	Rhizoma Alismatis
牡丹皮	mǔ dān pí	9g	Cortex Moutan
苍耳子	cāng ěr zǐ	9g	Fructus Xanthii
地肤子	dì fū zǐ	9g	Fructus Kochiae
麻子仁	má zǐ rén	9g	Fructus Cannabis
茯苓	fú líng	6g	Poria

Decoct in water. One dose per day for 7 days.

External Use: *Qū Shī Gāo* (祛湿膏)

【Second Visit】

After one week the itchiness was relieved, with less desquamation and crusting. The decoction was given again but modified with *shú dì huáng* (Radix Rehmanniae Praeparata) 15g and *dān shēn* (Radix et Rhizoma Salviae Miltiorrhizae) 9g. After 7 doses, the affected area completely healed and the itchiness was relieved.

Comments:

This clinical case was based on the pattern of heat in the muscles invaded by wind. Wind in the muscles for long periods of time can impair yin and exhaust blood. Herbs were prescribed to nourish yin, clear heat, moisten dryness, and relieve itchiness. Treatment lasted for over one month, after which the entire condition was resolved.

(Guang An Men Hospital of China Academy of Chinese Medical Sciences. *Clinical Experience Recordings of Zhu Ren-kang* (朱仁康临床经验集). Beijing: The People's Medical Publishing House, 1994, 231)

3. Case Studies of Xuan Guo-wei: Damp-heat and Blood Heat

Mr. Liu, 29 years old.

【Initial Visit】

Feb 25th, 1996. Mr. Liu's hair had been falling out for the past 3 years. His hair began to rapidly fall out with manifestations of oily hair, excessive dandruff, and itchiness. Severe hair loss also occurred when he didn't sleep enough or experienced too much stress. Much of his hair fell out whenever he washed or combed his hair. There was no hair on the forehead and vertex. He reported a sensation of heat on his head, insomnia, profuse dreams, soreness and weakness in the lower back and knees, and profuse nocturia.

Examination: Most of the hair on the forehead and temporal regions had fallen out completely. The anterior hair line was further back, with the forehead appearing higher. Head hair appeared thin, soft, dry, and short. The affected regions on the scalp appeared shiny. Red tongue, white thick greasy coating, and a wiry, slippery pulse.

【Pattern Differentiation】

Damp-heat accumulation, blood heat blocking the channels and collaterals.

【Treatment Principle】

Drain dampness, clear heat, eliminate fat, cool blood, unblock the channels and collaterals, and regrow hair.

【Prescription】

蒲公英	pú gōng yīng	30g	Herba Taraxaci
玄参	xuán shēn	20g	Radix Scrophulariae
生地黄	shēng dì huáng	20g	Radix Rehmanniae
丹参	dān shēn	20g	Radix et Rhizoma Salviae Miltiorrhizae
牡丹皮	mǔ dān pí	20g	Cortex Moutan
白花蛇舌草	bái huā shé shé cǎo	20g	Herba Hedyotis Diffusae
崩大碗	bēng dà wǎn	15g	Herba Centellae
女贞子	nǚ zhēn zǐ	15g	Fructus Ligustri Lucidi
茵陈蒿	yīn chén	15g	Herba Artemisiae Scopariae
侧柏叶	cè bǎi yè	15g	Cacumen Platycladi
蔓荆子	màn jīng zǐ	15g	Fructus Viticis
桑叶	sāng yè	10g	Folium Mori
甘草	gān cǎo	5g	Radix et Rhizoma Glycyrrhizae

External Use: Apply *Qū Zhī Shēng Fà Dīng* (祛脂生发酊) on the affected area with *Zhī Yì Xìng Xǐ Yè B* (脂溢性洗液 B) as an external wash.

【Second Visit】

After taking the oral medicine for one month, the scalp itchiness and oiliness improved, and less hair fell out. The sensation of heat disappeared and his sleep had also returned back to normal. However, he still complained of a sore and weak lower back and knees, and profuse nocturia. The former prescription was applied with modifications. *Màn jīng zǐ* (Fructus Viticis), *yīn chén* (Herba Artemisiae Scopariae), and *bái huā shé shé cǎo* (Herba Hedyotis Diffusae) were removed, and *sāng jì shēng* (Herba Taxilli) 15g, *shān zhū yú* (Fructus Corni) 10g, *jīn yīng zǐ* (Fructus

Rosae Laevigatae) 15g, and *zhì hé shǒu wū* (Radix Polygoni Multiflori Praeparata cum Succo Glycines Sotae) 15g were added.

【Third Visit】

After one month of treatment, hair loss became less prominent and the itchiness and oiliness disappeared. The symptoms of profuse nocturia and his sore, weak lower back and knees also significantly improved. Hair began to regrow in the vertex and frontal regions. After taking the medicine for another 2 months, hair grew up to 2 cm. The patient was then instructed to take oral liquids to consolidate the therapeutic effects and nourish hair. Six months later, his hair became healthy and beautiful once again.

(Xuan Guo-wei, Fan Rei-qiang, Chen Da-chan. Editors-in-chief. *Clinical Essence of Chinese Medicine Dermatology* (中医皮肤病临证精粹). Guangdong: Guangdong People's Publishing House, 2001, 147-148)

4. CASE STUDIES OF HU GUO-JUN: CONGEALING YIN COLD

Mr. Li, 24 years old.

【Initial Visit】

October 26th, 1984. The patient had suffered with phlegm in his body for quite a long time. He often coughed clear phlegm and felt cold, especially on his back. All of his symptoms had become aggravated since the autumn when his hair began to fall out, especially when he was combing his hair. One month later, his hair became very scant and thin. He then came in for medical treatment.

The patient appeared emaciated. His cough was aggravated, with the expectoration of clear phlegm. He complained of cold limbs and was averse to cold, especially on his back. His tongue was pale with a thin white coating. His pulses were deficient, thready, deep, and slow.

【Pattern Differentiation】

Congealing yin cold due to yang qi deficiency.

【Treatment Principle】

Warm yang and dissipate cold.

【Prescription】

鹿角片	lù jiǎo piàn	20g	Cornu Cervi
制附子	zhì fù zǐ	10g	Radix Aconiti Lateralis Praeparata
白芥子	bái jiè zǐ	10g	Semen Sinapis
桂枝	guì zhī	10g	Ramulus Cinnamomi
麻黄	má huáng	6g	Herba Ephedrae
细辛	xì xīn	6g	Radix et Rhizoma Asari
干姜	gān jiāng	6g	Rhizoma Zingiberis
熟地黄	shú dì huáng	30g	Radix Rehmanniae Praeparata
茯苓	fú líng	30g	Poria
紫石英	zǐ shí yīng	30g	Fluoritum (decoct first)

Decoct in water. One dose per day for 7 days.

【Second Visit】

After taking the prescription, the patient's cough was relieved. Symptoms of yin cold such as aversion to cold and the cold back improved a little, but the alopecia condition remained unchanged. The former prescription was applied with modifications. *Lù jiǎo piàn* (Cornu Cervi) was replaced with *lù jiǎo jiāo* (Colla Cornus Cervi) (decocted alone) 10g; *bái jiè zǐ* (Semen Sinapis) was decreased to 6g, *gān jiāng* (Rhizoma Zingiberis) to 3g; and added were *dāng guī* (Radix Angelicae Sinensis) 10g and *yín yáng huò* (Herba Epimedii) 20g. The patient was instructed to take the prescription for 3 months. The following spring, he stopped coughing completely and the condition of alopecia was also cured.

(Hu Guo-jun. Analysis of Alopecia Syndromes (脱发证治初探). *New Chinese Medicine* (新中医), 1991, (10): 10)

5. Case Studies of Bai Ya-ping: Weak Nutritive Qi and Strong Defensive Qi

Mr. Zhang, 32 years old.

【Initial Visit】

December 1999. The patient complained of itchiness, profuse dandruff, and a sensation of heat on his scalp for 6 years. In the previous 2 years, hair began falling from the temporal region to the vertex. Hair loss was more significant in the spring and summer. He also reported washing his hair with cold water.

Examination: fine and thin hair on the temporal regions and towards the vertex, excessive dandruff, red tongue, scant tongue coating, and a wiry, thready, and rapid pulse.

【Pattern Differentiation】

Weak nutritive qi and strong defensive qi.

【Treatment Principle】

Tonify the nutritive qi and quell the defensive qi.

【Prescription】

Modified *Guì Zhī Jiā Sháo Yào Tāng* (桂枝加芍药汤)

桂枝	guì zhī	9g	Ramulus Cinnamomi
白芍	bái sháo	9g	Radix Paeoniae Alba
桑叶	sāng yè	9g	Folium Mori
菊花	jú huā	9g	Flos Chrysanthemi
生甘草	shēng gān cǎo	6g	Radix et Rhizoma Glycyrrhizae
蝉蜕	chán tuì	6g	Periostracum Cicadae
生地黄	shēng dì huáng	12g	Radix Rehmanniae

Decoct with water, one dose per day.

【Second Visit】

The itching improved after 7 doses. He then took another 20 doses and the dandruff decreased significantly. Subsequently, he took the decoction every other day for 8 months. At this point, his hair had grown back; black in color and thick over the entire scalp.

(Bi Ya-jun, Lü Jin-cang, Liu Er-jun. 3 Cases of Treating Alopeica from the Nutritive and Defensive Qi (从营卫论治脱发验案 3 则). *New Journal* of Traditional Chinese Medicine (新中医). 2002, 34(10): 62)

6. Case Studies of Yu Wen-qiu: Yin Essence Deficiency, Spleen and Stomach Damp-heat

Mr. Yang, 25 years old.

【Initial Visit】

March 21, 2004. Mr. Yang's alopecia began half a year ago. It was particularly apparent to him early in the morning when he would find 20 to 30 pieces of hair on his pillow. He was bald on the temporal and vertex regions, and on other parts of his scalp his hair was thin, soft, and oily with excessive dandruff. Other symptoms included insomnia, poor appetite, a yellow greasy tongue coating, and a slippery rapid pulse.

【Pattern Differentiation】

Yin essence deficiency and damp-heat in the spleen and stomach.

【Treatment Principle】

Nourish yin and tonify blood, clear heat, and eliminate dampness.

【Prescription】

紫河车	zǐ hé chē	15g	Placenta Hominis (grind into powder and swallow with warm water)
仙茅	xiān máo	10g	Rhizoma Curculiginis
仙灵脾	xiān líng pí	10g	Herba Epimedii
女贞子	nǚ zhēn zǐ	15g	Fructus Ligustri Lucidi
旱莲草	hàn lián cǎo	15g	Herba Ecliptae
丹参	dān shēn	20g	Radix et Rhizoma Salviae Miltiorrhizae
侧柏叶	cè bǎi yè	10g	Cacumen Platycladi
藿香	huò xiāng	10g	Herba Agastachis
白花蛇舌草	bái huā shé shé cǎo	30g	Herba Hedyotis Diffusae
石菖蒲	shí chāng pú	10g	Rhizoma Acori Tatarinowii
黄柏	huáng bǎi	10g	Cortex Phellodendri Chinensis
知母	zhī mǔ	10g	Rhizoma Anemarrhenae
木瓜	mù guā	20g	Fructus Chaenomelis
合欢皮	hé huān pí	15g	Cortex Albiziae

【Second Visit】

On May 20, after 2 months of treatment, the alopecia had completely resolved. Hair had returned to the temporal and vertex regions, and his sleeping and appetite were also normal. The former prescription was continued with modifications. *Bái huā shé shé cǎo* (Herba Hedyotis Diffusae), *huáng bǎi* (Cortex Phellodendri Chinensis), and *zhī mǔ* (Rhizoma Anemarrhenae) were removed, and *pèi lán* (Herba Eupatorii) 10g, *huáng qí* (Radix Astragali) 30g, and *dāng guī* (Radix Angelicae Sinensis) 10g were added. After 3 months, healthy hair growth had returned.

(Ding Xiong-fei. Experience of Yu Wen-qiu in the Treatment of Seborrheic Alopecia (喻文球治疗脂溢性脱发经验). *Jiangxi Journal of Chinese Medicine* (江西中医药), 2005, 36(6): 7-8)

Discussions

1. Zhao Bing-nan: Two–Pattern Differentiates and Treatment of Androgenetic Alopecia

Zhao holds that androgenetic alopecia may be clinically differentiated into two general patterns. The first pattern is damp-heat. This pattern results from damp-heat accumulation in the interior combined with pathogenic wind invasion, resulting in damp-heat steaming the head and accumulating beneath the skin. This blocks the hair from receiving necessary nutrients.

The other pattern is blood dryness, manifesting with excessive dandruff, dry hair, fine and thin hair on the temporal and vertex regions of the head, and itchiness that is described as if insects were crawling on the scalp. This is caused by blood deficiency and wind dryness, which also leads to malnourishment of the hair.

To treat damp-heat alopecia, it is essential to strengthen the spleen, dispel dampness, course wind, and strengthen hair. Zhao uses *Qū Shī*

Jiàn Fà Tāng (祛湿健发汤) for damp-heat patterns. For blood dryness, it is important to apply medicinals that nourish blood, tonify yin, and darken hair color. He uses *Jù Shēng Zǐ Tāng* (苣胜子汤) for blood dryness patterns.

Different external washes are also used, depending on the presence of an oily, or dry-type alopecia.

➢ Oily Alopecia

| 透骨草 | tòu gǔ cǎo | 30g | Caulis Impatientis |
| 枯矾 | kū fán | 10g | Alumen dehydratum |

Decoct in water until 2000 ml of the liquid remains. Use the decoction as an external wash, 2-3 times every week.

➢ Dry Alopecia

【Prescription】

透骨草	tòu gǔ cǎo	20g	Caulis Impatientis
侧柏叶	cè bǎi yè	15g	Cacumen Platycladi
皂角刺	zào jiǎo cì	10g	Spina Gleditsiae

Decoct in water until 2000 ml remains. Use the decoction as an external wash, 1-2 times every week.

Both external wash prescriptions include *tòu gǔ cǎo* (Caulis Impatientis). Zhao says that this herb is acrid and warm, with functions to dispel wind, remove dampness, soothe the sinews, invigorate blood, and relieve pain. It may be taken orally to treat rheumatoid diseases, or can be used as an external wash for carbuncles. Zhao once experimented by adding this herb to an external wash to treat a seborrheic dermatitis patient with oily symptoms. He discovered that this herb was excellent at relieving itching and eliminating fat, so he continued to apply this herb for cases of oily alopecia.

(Qin Han-kun. Syndromes and Treatments for Alopecia (脱发证治). *Journal of Traditional Chinese Medicine* (中医杂志), 1986, (12): 10)

2. Chen Da-chan: Clinical Experience of Androgenetic Alopecia

(1) Differentiating Syndromes by Combining Deficiency and Excess Patterns

Through many years of clinical experience, Dr. Chen views androgenetic alopecia as being related to deficiencies of liver or kidney, as well as to excesses of dampness or heat. *Basic Questions—Five Zang Coming into Being* (素问·五脏生成篇, *Sù Wèn: Wǔ Zàng Shēng Chéng Piān*) says: "If one eats too much sweet, pain of the bones result, and hair falls out." The spleen dominates transformation and transportation. It is also the source of post-natal energy. An improper diet containing too much greasy, sweet, spicy, or fried food or alcohol leads to impairment of the spleen. The spleen will then lose its transformative and transportative functions, leading to water dampness accumulation. Dampness accumulation can linger for a long period, over time transforming into heat, thereby causing damp-heat. Dampness has a sticky nature; and heat naturally rises. Humid climates will aggravate damp-heat, both interiorly within the body and exteriorly; such that it will rise up to the head. Damp-heat can damage the integrity of the hair follicles and cause hair to become oily and ultimately fall out. This pattern is very difficult to treat.

(2) Strengthen the Kidney and Spleen while Clearing Heat and Eliminating Dampness

In clinic, Chen treats androgenic alopecia by tonifying the liver, kidney, and spleen, as well as the overall qi. Tonifying kidney essence also nourishes wood. Strengthening spleen qi also helps to produce blood. Tonifying the post-natal qi strengthens the congenital essence. He also aims to clear heat and eliminate dampness. The prescription *Liù Wèi Dì Huáng Wán* (六味地黄丸) plus *Èr Zhì Wán* (二至丸), and modified *Sì Jūn Zǐ Tāng* (四君子汤) are recommended for these purposes. The exact herbs are as follows: *huáng qí* (Radix Astragali), *gān dì huáng* (Radix Rehmanniae), *huái shān yào* (Rhizoma Dioscoreae), *tài zǐ shēn* (Radix Pseudostellariae), *nǚ zhēn zǐ* (Fructus Ligustri Lucidi), *hàn lián cǎo* (Herba Ecliptae), *zhì hé shǒu wū* (Radix Polygoni Multiflori Praeparata cum Succo Glycines Sotae), *yún fú líng* (Poriae), *zé xiè* (Rhizoma Alismatis), *bái zhú* (Rhizoma Atractylodis Macrocephalae), *dān shēn* (Radix et Rhizoma Salviae Miltiorrhizae), *pú gōng yīng* (Herba Taraxaci), and *gān cǎo* (Radix et Rhizoma Glycyrrhizae).

Analysis of the herbal prescription: *Huáng qí* (Radix Astragali) tonifies qi and strengthens the superficial level, while strengthening the hair follicles so that hair will not fall out. *Huái shān yào* (Rhizoma Dioscoreae), *tài zǐ shēn* (Radix Pseudostellariae), and *bái zhú* (Rhizoma Atractylodis Macrocephalae) strengthen spleen qi. The *Essentials of the Materia Medica* (*Běn Cǎo Bèi Yào*, 本草备要) says: "*Nǚ zhēn zǐ* (Fructus Ligustri Lucidi) can tonify liver and kidney, calm the five *zang* organs, strengthen the back and knees, brighten the eyes, and blacken hair color". *Grand Materia Medica* (*Běn Cǎo Gāng Mù*, 本草纲目) says: "*Hàn lián cǎo* (Herba Ecliptae) can blacken hair color and tonify kidney yin."Both *nǚ zhēn zǐ* (Fructus Ligustri Lucidi) and *hàn lián cǎo* (Herba Ecliptae) work together to tonify liver and kidney yin. *Hé shǒu wū* (Radix Polygoni Multiflori) tonifies the liver and kidney, tonifies blood and essence, and darkens hair color. *Yún fú líng* (Poriae) and *zé xiè* (Rhizoma Alismatis) act to strengthen the spleen and remove dampness. These 2 herbs have the ability to clear excess and tonify without causing stagnation. *Gān dì huáng* (Radix Rehmanniae) and *dān shēn* (Radix et Rhizoma Salviae Miltiorrhizae) can clear heat, cool blood, and move blood. *Pú gōng yīng* (Herba Taraxaci) can clear heat, remove dampness, and eliminate hair oiliness. *Pú gōng yīng* (Herba Taraxaci) can prevent the herbal prescription from becoming too warm, which may impair yin and blood. *Gān cǎo* (Radix et Rhizoma Glycyrrhizae) tonifies spleen qi and harmonizes all the herbs in the prescription. All the herbs work together to tonify the liver, kidney, qi and blood; clear heat, remove dampness, and help hair to regrow.

For excessive sebaceous gland secretions, which is a damp-heat type of alopecia, add *tŭ fú líng* (Rhizoma Smilacis Glabrae), *yīn chén* (Herba Artemisiae Scopariae), *shān zhā* (Fructus Crataegi), *bù zhā yè* (Microcoris Folium), *bái huā shé shé cǎo* (Herba Hedyotis Diffusae), or *bēng dà wǎn* (Herba Centellae) to clear heat, eliminate dampness.

When the scalp is very itchy, add *bái xiān pí* (Cortex Dictamni), *dì fū zǐ* (Fructus Kochiae), and *jiāng cán* (Bombyx Batryticatus) to expel wind and relieve itching.

If the hair is dry and yellow with dandruff caused by a blood deficiency/heat and wind dryness, add *bái sháo* (Radix Paeoniae Alba), *chì sháo* (Radix Paeoniae Rubra), *dān pí* (Cortex Moutan), *dāng guī* (Radix Angelicae Sinensis), *yì mǔ cǎo* (Herba Leonuri), *jī xuè téng* (Caulis Spatholobi), *zǐ cǎo* (Radix Arnebiae), *bái jí lí* (Fructus Tribuli), and *cè bǎi yè* (Cacumen Platycladi) to nourish blood, expel wind, and nourish dryness.

If the patient has soreness and pain in the lower back and knees with nocturia, add *gǒu qǐ zǐ* (Fructus Lycii), *tù sī zǐ* (Semen Cuscutae), *huái niú xī* (Radix Achyranthis Bidentatae), *sāng jì shēng* (Herba Taxilli), *huáng jīng* (Rhizoma Polygonati), and *shān yú ròu* (Fructus Corni) to tonify the liver and kidney, and tonify essence and blood.

If the patient has vexation, thirst, mouth ulcers, a red tongue with a scant tongue coating and a thready rapid pulse (which is yin deficiency and excessive fire), add *sāng shèn* (Fructus Mori), *zhī mǔ* (Rhizoma Anemarrhenae), *huáng bǎi* (Cortex Phellodendri Chinensis), and *xuán shēn* (Radix Scrophulariae) to nourish yin, clear heat, and expel fire.

If the patient has stress, insomnia, and profuse dreaming, add *mǔ lì* (Concha Ostreae), *lóng chǐ* (Dens Dragonis), *yè jiāo téng* (Caulis Polygoni Multiflori), *hé huān pí* (Cortex Albiziae), and *suān zǎo rén* (Semen Ziziphi

Spinosae) to calm the spirit and relieve depression.

(3) To nourish hair, use large dosages of *huáng qí* (Radix Astragali) and *dān shēn* (Radix et Rhizoma Salviae Miltiorrhizae)

"Qi is the command of blood". Qi produces blood, moves blood, and controls blood. Professor Chen believes that between qi and blood, qi is more important in regards to the health of hair. Sufficient qi can increase the production of blood, and therefore can help strengthen and grow hair. In clinic, many alopecia patients enter the clinic with qi deficiency symptoms such as fatigue, easily getting tired, spontaneous sweating, and a thready, weak pulse. Herbs that tonify the liver and kidney, nourish blood, or move blood tend to work too slowly. However, using *huáng qí* (Radix Astragali) in large dosages can tonify qi to produce blood very effectively. Modern pharmacological researches have demonstrated that *huáng qí* (Radix Astragali) regulates the immune system, dilates blood vessels and regulates blood circulation. It can also help the hair to regrow. Its main ingredient is calycosin, which has an antagonistic function to androgen.

Modern research has shown that alopecia patients have problems with poor circulation. This is mainly manifested by sluggish blood circulation and viscous blood. Dr. Chen believes that by adding herbs that improve blood circulation and remove blood stasis such as *dān shēn* (Radix et Rhizoma Salviae Miltiorrhizae), microcirculation is improved and thus more nutrients reach the hair follicles. Its active ingredient, tanshinone, has shown estrogen-like characteristics and anti-androgenic effects, which also benefits the immune system. It also serves as an anti-bacterial agent with the ability to eliminate oils.

(Liu Wei. Clinic Experience of Professor Chen Da-can in the Treatment of Seborrheic Alopecia (陈达灿教授论治脂溢性脱发经验撷萃). *Chinese Archives of Traditional Chinese Medicine* (中医药学刊). 2004, 22(1): 10-11)

3. Yu Wen-Qiu: Treatment of Androgenetic Alopecia

In Yu's theory, the origin of alopecia lies in yin essence deficiency and unconsolidated essence qi, with wind disturbing upwards. Its manifestations appear as blood heat, wind dryness, and damp heat in the spleen and stomach. This rationale comes from fundamental theories such as "The kidney stores essence, and is manifested in the hair", "hair is the effulgence of the blood", and "essence and blood transform into each other". Patients may have patterns of damp-heat in the spleen and stomach but they may also have kidney essence deficiency, thereby holding both patterns of excess and deficiency. The general principle is to tonify yin essence without draining the essence of the hair, move blood circulation, and remove blood stasis. The achievements of modern research are also used to treat alopecia. The basic prescription is as follows:

(1) *Shén Yìng #1 Shēng Fà Tāng* (神应 I 号生发汤)

Shén Yìng #1 Shēng Fà Tāng is indicated for dry androgenic alopecia: *zǐ hé chē* (Placenta Hominis) (powdered) 15g, *xiān máo* (Rhizoma Curculiginis) 10g, *xiān líng pí* (Herba Epimedii) 10g, *nǚ zhēn zǐ* (Fructus Ligustri Lucidi) 15g, *hàn lián cǎo* (Herba Ecliptae) 15g, *sāng shèn* (Fructus Mori) 30g, *shǒu wū téng* (Caulis Polygoni Multiflori) 20g, *jī xuè téng* (Caulis Spatholobi) 20g, *hóng huā* (Flos Carthami) 15g, *mù guā* (Fructus Chaenomelis) 20g, *shí chāng pú* (Rhizoma Acori Tatarinowii) 15g, *huáng qí* (Radix Astragali) 30g, *bái zhú* (dry-fried Rhizoma Atractylodis Macrocephalae) 10g, and *cè bǎi yè* (Cacumen Platycladi) 10g.

Zǐ hé chē (Placenta Hominis) tonifies essence, nourishes blood, and tonifies qi. Modern research has demonstrated that it contains estrogens. *Xiān máo* (Rhizoma Curculiginis), *xiān líng pí* (Herba Epimedii), *Èr Zhì Wán*, and *sāng shèn* (Fructus Mori) tonify kidney essence and expel wind. They all serve as the chief medicinals in this formula. *Shǒu wū téng* (Caulis Polygoni Multiflori), *jī xuè téng* (Caulis Spatholobi), and *hóng huā* (Flos Carthami) tonify blood, move blood, expel wind, and dredge the hair roots. They serve as the deputy medicinals. *Mù guā* (Fructus Chaenomelis) and *shí chāng pú* (Rhizoma Acori) eliminate stagnation from the tonifying herbs, free the collaterals, and open the orifices. They serve as the assistant and envoy herbs. *Huáng qí* (Radix Astragali) and *bái zhú* (dry-fried Rhizoma Atractylodis Macrocephalae) strengthen the spleen and generate blood. They serve as the assistant herbs. *Huáng qí* (Radix Astragali) also have amino acids which can increase estrogen levels. Dr. Yu has clinical experience using *cè bǎi yè* (Cacumen Platycladi) to clear out oiliness and regrow hair.

(2) *Shén Yìng #2 Shēng Fà Tāng* (神应 II 号生发汤)

Shén Yìng #2 Shēng Fà Tāng is indicated for damp androgenetic alopecia: *zǐ hé chē* (Placenta Hominis) (powdered) 15g, *xiān máo* (Rhizoma Curculiginis) 10g, *xiān líng pí* (Herba Epimedii) 10g, *nǚ zhēn zǐ* (Fructus Ligustri Lucidi) 15g, *hàn lián cǎo* (Herba Ecliptae) 15g, *dān shēn* (Radix et Rhizoma Salviae Miltiorrhizae) 20g, *chì sháo* (Radix Paeoniae Rubra) 15g, *huò xiāng* (Herba Agastachis) 10g, *pèi lán* (Herba Eupatorii) 10g, *bái huā shé shé cǎo* (Herba Hedyotis Diffusae) 30g, *mù guā* (Fructus Chaenomelis) 20g, *qín jiāo* (Radix Gentianae Macrophyllae) 12g, *huáng qí* (raw Radix Astragali) 30g, *bái zhú* (dry-fried Rhizoma Atractylodis Macrocephalaed) 10g, and *fáng fēng* (Radix Saposhnikoviae) 10g.

In the formula, *dān shēn* (Radix et Rhizoma Salviae Miltiorrhizae) and *chì sháo* (Radix Paeoniae Rubra) nourish, move, and cool the blood. *Huò xiāng* (Herba Agastachis) and *pèi lán* (Herba Eupatorii) are acrid and neutral, which transform dampness and arouse the spleen without impairing the stomach. *Bái huā shé shé cǎo* (Herba Hedyotis Diffusae) drains damp-heat, utilizing the principle of "acrid herbs release, and bitter herbs drain downward". *Mù guā* (Fructus Chaenomelis) and *qín jiāo* (Radix Gentianae Macrophyllae) clear deficient heat, dispel wind, free the channels and collaterals, and open the orifices. *Fáng fēng* (Radix Saposhnikoviae) is a wind-expelling medicinal which is of a moist nature. It can expel both exterior and interior wind without detrimental effects to the hair.

(3) External Treatment

A. *Wài Xǐ I Hào* (外洗 I 号) is for dry androgenic alopecia: *sāng yè* (Folium Mori) 30g, *má yè* (Cannabis Folium) 30g, *lù lù tōng* (Fructus Liquidambaris) 30g, *cè bǎi yè* (Cacumen Platycladi) 30g, *tòu gǔ pí* (Caulis Impatientis) 30g, and *shǒu wū* (Radix Polygoni Multiflori) 30g.

B. *Wài Xǐ II Hào* is for damp androgenic alopecia: *tǔ fú líng* (Rhizoma Smilacis Glabrae) 30g, *yín huā* (Caulis Lonicerae Japonicae) 30g, *wáng bù liú xíng* (Semen Vaccariae) 30g, *tòu gǔ cǎo* (Caulis Impatientis) 30g, *zào jiǎo* (Spina Gleditsiae) 30g, and *hòu pò* (Cortex Magnoliae Officinalis) 15g.

(Ding Xiong-fei. Yu Wen-qiu's Experience of Seborrheic Alopecia Treatment (喻文球治疗脂溢性脱发经验). *Jiangxi Journal of Traditional Chinese Medicine* (江西中医药), 2005, 36(6): 7-8)

PERSPECTIVES OF INTEGRATIVE MEDICINE

Challenges and Solutions

Androgenic alopecia is associated with hair falling out mainly from the forehead, temporal, and vertex regions, usually beginning in adolescence. With chronic long-term alopecia, it is often difficult to cure because the hair follicle can no longer be nourished due to atrophic degeneration. Therefore, the goal in this case is to control alopecia, delay its progression, and improve the conditions for regrowing new hair.

Challenge #1: How to Control Alopecia

The course of androgenic alopecia is similar to that of alopecia areata. Androgenic alopecia has an active stage and dormant stage. In the active stage, the determining factor and prognosis lies in how much hair is falling out during this stage. At this stage, it is important to put a strong focus on treatment on controlling hair loss. In the clinic, it is essential to place attention to the following points:

Medical treatment: Chinese medicine and biomedicines should be combined. It is still imperative to emphasize pattern differentiation and treatment, however. Endocrine function must be regulated by addressing the balance of yin and yang. Although steroids are very often used to treat severe cases of alopecia, their side effects should be seriously considered.

Alopecia can worsen if its related symptoms are not controlled; such as sebum secretion, itching, and desquamation. Managing these symptoms can improve most alopecia conditions. Treatment should focus on internal medical interventions and external lifestyle patterns. Patients need to improve their diet, regulate sleep, and manage stress.

Challenge #2: How to Decrease the Sebum Secretion

Hypersteatosis is the main symptom of androgenic alopecia. Decreasing the secretion of sebum improves alopecia conditions. Hypersteatosis is the manifestation of a metabolic disorder and systemic endocrine dysfunction. For treatment, herbs are used both as an internal medicine and as an exterior herbal wash.

For internal medicine, treatment is focused on the root, to decrease sebum secretions with herbs such as *shān zhā* (Fructus Crataegi), *mài yá* (Fructus Hordei Germinatus), *chì shí zhī* (Halloysitum Rubrum), *pú gōng yīng* (Herba Taraxaci), *cè bǎi yè* (Cacumen Platycladi), *sāng yè* (Folium

Mori), *bù zhā yè* (Microcoris Folium), and *zhì hé shǒu wū* (Radix Polygoni Multiflori Praeparata cum Succo Glycines Sotae).

The external wash also decreases sebum secretion by using herbs such as *liú huáng* (Sulfur), *cè bǎi yè* (Cacumen Platycladi), *tòu gǔ cǎo* (Caulis Impatientis), *wáng bù liú xíng* (Semen Vaccariae), *zào jiǎo cì* (Spina Gleditsiae), and *xiān hè cǎo* (Herba Agrimoniae).

CHALLENGE #3: HOW TO IMPROVE HAIR GROWTH

Hair growth typically displays three cycles. With alopecia, the patients' hair is usually fine and brittle. Most of these patients' hair stopped growing during the early stages. The scalp generally develops a bright and shiny appearance with only a few brittle hairs. The hair follicle will also have become atrophied. At this point, the disease will be hard to cure, and hair transplantation is suggested in these cases. The number of hair follicles on the human head is limited, so the focus is to stop the disease from progressing, improve the conditions to promote hair growth, and prevent the hair follicle from atrophy. Both internal medicine and external treatments are applied. For the interior treatment, the focus is to inhibit androgens, enzyme activities, and modulate androgen receptors by using Chinese herbs that tonify the kidney and move blood. For the external treatment, topical herbal formulations concentrate the medicine on the affected areas of the scalp and also reduce the side effects of drugs. Plum blossom needles can also stimulate the scalp and promote hair growth.

Insight from Empirical Wisdom

Androgenetic alopecia is one of the difficult diseases to treat in dermatology, particularly when stimulating hair regeneration. As living standards have improved and people are able to afford the means to improve their aesthetic appearance, more people actively seek treatment for alopecia. In order to improve this condition, attention should be placed on the following points:

1. MODIFICATIONS ACCORDING TO CHANGES IN THE SYNDROME

There are numerous causes for alopecia, its clinical manifestations, and the various accompanying symptoms. The treatments for each person will vary, depending on the presenting syndrome differentiation. Treating the source of the problem is necessary to cure the condition.

【Modifications】

➢ If the patient has oily dandruff and red scalp lesions, add *bái zhǐ* (Radix Angelicae Dahuricae), *yì yǐ rén* (Semen Coicis), and *chì shí zhī* (Halloysitum Rubrum) to clear heat, transform dampness, and astringe the oiliness.

➢ If the patient has severe insomnia, add *zhū shā* (Cinnabaris), *cí shí* (Magnetitum), and *zhēn zhū mǔ* (Concha Margaritifera) to calm the mind.

➢ If the patient has a distending pain in the chest and hypochondria, add *chuān liàn zǐ* (Fructus Toosendan), *yù jīn* (Radix Curcumae), and *zhǐ qiào* (Fructus Aurantii) to smooth the liver qi, resolve constraint, and relieve pain.

➢ If the patient has itchiness, add *bái xiān pí* (Cortex Dictamni), *jiāng cán* (Bombyx Batryticatus), and *suān zǎo rén* (Semen Ziziphi Spinosae) to expel wind, calm the mind, and relieve itching.

➢ If the patient has obvious qi stagnation and blood stasis, add *táo rén* (Semen Persicae), *chuān xiōng* (Rhizoma Chuanxiong), *yì mǔ cǎo* (Herba Leonuri), and *cè bǎi yè* (Cacumen Platycladi) to invigorate blood and transform stasis.

➢ If the patient has blood deficiency, add *dāng guī* (Radix Angelicae Sinensis), *bái sháo* (Radix Paeoniae Alba), and *shú dì huáng* (Radix Rehmanniae Praeparata).

2. Insight for Treatment and Medicinal Application

Alopecia is related to blood disease. In biomedicine, alopecia is related to high levels of blood coagulation. After many failed courses of treatment for chronic alopecia, blood stasis conditions may have been overlooked. Using methods to invigorate blood and transform stasis can be effective at growing new hair.

The herbs to treat this type of blood stasis in alopecia are: *yì mǔ cǎo* (Herba Leonuri), *dān shēn* (Radix et Rhizoma Salviae Miltiorrhizae), *mǔ dān pí* (Cortex Moutan), *shēng dì huáng* (Radix Rehmanniae), *guàn zhòng* (Cyrtomii Rhizoma), *cè bǎi yè* (Cacumen Platycladi), *táo rén* (Semen Persicae), and *hóng huā* (Flos Carthami). Herbs that are bitter and drying are to be avoided because they can impair yin and blood.

Other herbs can be utilized to heal alopecia for different syndromes. Herbs that clear heat can help with alopecia such as *pú gōng yīng* (Herba Taraxaci), *mǔ dān pí* (Cortex Moutan), and *shēng dì huáng* (Radix Rehmanniae). Most alopecia patients have a hot constitution with exogenous pathogens attacking the body at the hair and orifices.

Grand Materia Medica (本草纲目 , *Běn Cǎo Gāng Mù*) says: "*Pú gōng yīng* (Herba Taraxaci) can darken the hair and strengthen the tendons and bones". In modern pharmacology, *pú gōng yīng* (Herba Taraxaci) is known to contain inose, which helps hair growth. Most herbal medicines for alopecia are warm. When combined with *pú gōng yīng* (Herba Taraxaci), their warm and dry properties could be counterbalanced so as not to impair yin fluids and blood essence.

Because alopecia patients typically display higher levels of lead, herbs such as *kūn bù* (Thallus Laminariae) and *hǎi zǎo* (Sargassum) can resolve toxins to eliminate lead, invigorate blood and dissipate nodules to grow hair.

For excessive sebum secretions, add *hé shǒu wū* (Radix Polygoni

Multiflori), *chì shí zhī* (Halloysitum Rubrum), *shān zhā* (Fructus Crataegi), *mài yá* (Fructus Hordei Germinatus), *bù zhā yè* (Microcoris Folium), and *cè bǎi yè* (Cacumen Platycladi) to control seborrhea. External herbal washes can be used as well. After the symptoms improve, medicinals can be added to strengthen the hair.

3. Combining Internal and External Treatment

Using a holistic approach, syndrome differentiation, and regulation of the whole body, internal treatments can treat the root of the problem. External treatment can treat the branch by focusing on the local affected areas. Both methods are effective in enhancing the treatments for both the interior and exterior, both the root and branch. When using the external liniment, it is more effective if the hair is shaved.

For external application, *Wū Fà Shēng Fà Dīng* (乌发生发酊), *Qū Zhī Shēng Fà Dīng* (祛脂生发酊), *Zhǐ Yǎng Shēng Fà Dīng* (止痒生发酊), and *Yì Fà B Wài Yòng Dīng* (益发 B 外用酊) are used. *Wū Fà Shēng Fà Dīng* (乌发生发酊) contains *biān tiáo shēn* (Radix Ginseng) and *xī yáng shēn* (Radix Panacis Quinquefolii), which provides nutrients for hair growth. It is mainly used to improve hair growth in cases of androgenic alopecia. *Yì Fà B Wài Yòng Dīng* (益发 B 外用酊) has *rén shēn yè* (Folium Ginseng), *huā jiāo* (Pericarpium Zanthoxyli), and *chuān xiōng* (Rhizoma Chuanxiong). *Rén shēn yè* (Folium Ginseng) has ingredients similar to *rén shēn* (Radix Ginseng) which stimulates the brain cortex, increases metabolism, prevents androgenic alopecia, and mimics estrogen function to counter androgen effects. *Huā jiāo* (Pericarpium Zanthoxyli), *chuān xiōng* (Rhizoma Chuanxiong), *dān shēn* (Radix et Rhizoma Salviae Miltiorrhizae), *chì sháo* (Radix Paeoniae Rubra), *cè bǎi yè* (Cacumen Platycladi), and *dāng guī* (Radix Angelicae Sinensis) invigorate blood and transform stasis. These herbs can stimulate hair follicles, dilate blood capillaries, promote microcirculation, increase nutrients to the hair follicles, and improve hair growth.

4. Adherence to Treatment

Hair loss is a hard condition to treat, and hair growth is a slow and long course. An immediate result from a brief course of treatment is not realistic. In the middle and latter stages of alopecia, results are even harder to attain. The key for success is strict adherence to the treatment plan. As long as the hair follicle has not been injured, hair can still grow.

Summary

Combining Chinese medicine and biomedicines can effectively treat and also prevent alopecia. The biomedical research on androgenic alopecia provides a deeper scientific foundation for the Chinese medicine system of clinical syndromes and treatment. The highest benefits occur by taking Chinese medicine internally while applying biomedicines externally. Regardless of which type of medicine (Chinese medicine or biomedicine), patients must adhere to the treatment plan for a long period of time. Internal and external remedies are recommended in the early and middle stages. Hair transplantation is recommended for the later stages of alopecia.

The focus of research is primarily on the mechanism of action of Chinese herbal medicine, the selection of Chinese herbal prescriptions for androgenic alopecia, and the development of safer and more effective medicinals.

SELECTED QUOTES FROM CLASSICAL TEXTS

Basic Questions—Treatise of Heavenly Truth from Remote Antiquity (素问·上古天真论, *Sù Wèn: Shàng Gǔ Tiān Zhēn Lùn*)

"女子七岁，肾气盛，齿更发长。……四七，筋骨坚，发长极。身体盛壮。五七，阳明脉衰，面始焦，发始堕。六七，三阳脉衰于上，面皆焦，发始白。" "丈夫八岁，皮肤气实，发长齿更。……三八，肾气平均，筋骨劲强，故真牙生而长极。……五八，肾气衰，发堕齿槁，六八，阳气衰竭于上，面焦，发鬓颁白。……八八，则齿发去。"

"When females are seven, the kidney will be abundant, and the teeth will grow. At age twenty eight, the tendons become strong, hair grows to its fullest, and the body is strong. At age thirty-five, the *yangming* channel declines, and the face begins to turn sallow, and the hair begins to fall out. At age forty-two, the three *yang* channels decline and its manifestations are reflected upwards: the face becomes sallow and the hair turns white."

"When males are eight, qi is abundant on the skin, as hair starts to grow, and teeth begin to change. At age twenty four, kidney qi is moderate, the tendons and bones are strong, and the teeth grow to their fullest. At age forty, as the kidney declines, the hair starts to fall out and the teeth start to wither. At age forty eight, *yang* qi declines and manifests upwards as the face becomes sallow and the hair becomes white. At age sixty four, the teeth and hair start to fall out."

Basic Questions—Five Zang Coming into Being (Sù Wèn: Wǔ Zàng Shēng Chén Piān 素问·五脏生成篇)

"其主脾也，是故……多食甘，则骨痛而发落。"

"The spleen governs, so eating too much sweet food will lead to pain in the bones and hair falling out."

Medical Bank Stone—Hair (Yī Biǎn: Xū Fà, 医碥·须发)

"年少发白早落，或头起白屑者，血热太过也。世俗只知发者血之余，以为血衰，不知血热发反不茂，火多血少，木反不荣，火至于顶，炎上之甚也。"

"If at a young age, the hair is white or falling out or there is dandruff on scalp, this is due to excessive blood heat. Hair is the manifestation of blood. While hair problems can be due to blood deficiency, most people do not realize that it can also be due to blood heat. When there is excessive fire with blood deficiency, wood cannot be nourished and fire will rise up to the head and stir."

Complete Book of Patterns and Treatments in External Medicine (外科证治全书 , *Wài Kē Zhèng Zhì Quán Shū*)

"蛀发癣，头上渐升秃斑，久则运开，干枯作痒，由阴虚热盛，剃头时风邪袭于孔腠，搏聚不散，血气不潮而成。而生木鳖切片浸数日，入锅煮豆煎汤，剃头后洗之，搽蜈蚣油，至愈乃止。又法：用草乌连皮切片，炙脆研粉，醋调，日涂三次，数日愈。"

"Long term tinea capitis will turn into alopecia areata. If tine capitis lasts for a long period of time, it will be dry and itchy because yin is deficient and heat is excessive. When cutting the hair, pathogenic wind attacks the pores and accumulates around there. Therefore, the hair could not be nourished by blood and qi. Cut *shēng mù biē* (Semen Momordicae) into pieces and put them into water, and several days later, cook it with beans. After cutting the hair, wash the scalp with this soup and put centipede oil on it, it will be cured. Another method is to cut *cǎo wū* (Radix Aconiti Kusnezoffii) into pieces with the peel, liquid-fry it, grind it into powder, and mix it with vinegar. Apply the mixture to the scalp three times a day, and it will be cured after several days of treatment."

Discussion of Blood Patterns—Blood Stasis (*Xuè Zhèng Lùn:·Yū Xuè*, 血证论·瘀血)

"瘀血在上焦，或发脱不生。"

"If blood stasis is located in upper *jiao*, it will lead to alopecia."

MODERN RESEARCH

Clinical Research

1. Pattern Differentiation and Corresponding Treatment

(1) Zhu Ren-kang divides alopecia into four types:

1) Blood heat and wind dryness

It should be treated by cooling blood, dispelling wind, relieving itching, and nourishing dryness. Herbal medicines are *shēng dì huáng* (Radix Rehmanniae), *shú dì huáng* (Radix Rehmanniae Praeparata), *hé shǒu wū* (Radix Polygoni Multiflori), *dāng guī* (Radix Angelicae Sinensis), *mǔ dān pí* (Cortex Moutan), *huǒ má rén* (Fructus Cannabis), *jí lí* (Fructus Tribuli), and *zhì gān cǎo* (Radix et Rhizoma Glycyrrhizae Praeparata cum Melle).

2) Damp-heat accumulating upwards

It should be treated by clearing damp-heat with modified *Lóng Dǎn Xiè Gān Tāng* (龙胆泻肝汤). Herbal medicines are *lóng dǎn cǎo* (Radix et Rhizoma Gentianae), *zé xiè* (Rhizoma Alismatis), *chē qián zǐ* (Semen Plantaginis), *huáng qín* (Radix Scutellariae), *shān zhā* (raw Fructus Crataegi), and *zhī zǐ* (raw Fructus Gardeniae).

3) Blood deficiency with wind dryness

It should be treated by nourishing blood and dryness with modified *Shén Yìng Yǎng Zhēn Dān* (神应养真丹).

Herbal medicines are *shú dì huáng* (Radix Rehmanniae Praeparata), *hé shǒu wū* (Radix Polygoni Multiflori), *dāng guī* (Radix Angelicae Sinensis), *dān shēn* (Radix et Rhizoma Salviae Miltiorrhizae), *tù sī zǐ* (Semen Cuscutae), *jí lí* (Fructus Tribuli), and *huáng qí* (Radix Astragali).

4) Liver and kidney deficiency

It should be treated by tonifying the liver and kidney with modified *Qī Bǎo Měi Rán Dān* (七宝美髯丹).

Herbal medicines are *shēng dì huáng* (Radix Rehmanniae), *shú dì huáng* (Radix Rehmanniae Praeparata), *fú líng* (Poria), *zé xiè* (Rhizoma Alismatis), *hé shǒu wū* (Radix Polygoni Multiflori), *shān zhū yú* (Fructus Corni), *nǚ zhēn zǐ* (Fructus Ligustri Lucidi), *hēi zhī ma* (Semen Sesami Nigrum), *hàn lián cǎo* (Herba Ecliptae), *yín yáng huò* (Herba Epimedii), and *xiān máo* (Rhizoma Curculiginis).[1]

(2) Chen Da-chan divides alopecia into three types:

1) Blood heat and wind dryness

It should be treated by cooling blood, clearing heat, dispelling wind, nourishing dryness with *shēng dì huáng* (Radix Rehmanniae) 15g, *jú huā* (Flos Chrysanthemi) 12g, *bái huā shé shé cǎo* (Herba Hedyotis Diffusae) 20g, *bái xiān pí* (Cortex Dictamni) 12g, *fáng fēng* (Radix Saposhnikoviae) 9g, *zǐ cǎo* (Radix Arnebiae) 12g, *bēng dà wǎn* (Herba Centellae) 15g, and *gān cǎo* (Radix et Rhizoma Glycyrrhizae) 6g.

2) Damp-heat accumulating upwards

It should be treated by clearing damp-heat. The prescription is *Yì Fà I Hào Fāng* (益发Ⅰ号方): *yīn chén* (Herba Artemisiae Scopariae) 15g, *chì shí zhī* (Halloysitum Rubrum) 15g, *bái xiān pí* (Cortex Dictamni)15g, *pú gōng yīng* (Herba Taraxaci) 20g, *shēng dì huáng* (Radix Rehmanniae) 9g, *bì xiè* (Rhizoma Dioscoreae Hypoglaucae) 12g, *bái zhú* (Rhizoma Atractylodis Macrocephalae) 9g, *shān zhā* (Fructus Crataegi) 20g, *bēng dà wǎn* (Herba Centellae) 20g, and *gān cǎo* (Radix et Rhizoma Glycyrrhizae) 6g.

3) Liver and kidney deficiency

It should be treated by tonifying the liver and kidney, nourishing hair and helping to regrow hair. The prescription is *Yì Fà III Hào Fāng* (益发Ⅲ号方): *hé shǒu wū* (Radix Polygoni Multiflori) 15g, *tù sī zǐ* (Semen Cuscutae) 18g, *gǒu qǐ zǐ* (Fructus Lycii) 9g, *hàn lián cǎo* (Herba Ecliptae) 15g, *yín yáng huò* (Herba Epimedii) 9g, *dǎng shēn* (Radix Codonopsis) 12g, and *zhì gān cǎo* (Radix et Rhizoma Glycyrrhizae Praeparata cum Melle) 6g.

If there is yin deficiency, then we can combine tonifying of the liver and kidney, nourishing yin to clear heat, and blackening and growing hair. The prescription is *Yì Fà II Hào Fāng* (益发Ⅱ号方): *pú gōng yīng* (Herba Taraxaci) 18g, *bēng dà wǎn* (Herba Centellae) 15g, *sāng shèn* (Fructus Mori) 15g, *nǚ zhēn zǐ* (Fructus Ligustri Lucidi) 18g, *hàn lián cǎo* (Herba

Ecliptae) 18g, *hé shǒu wū* (Radix Polygoni Multiflori) 15g, *bái zhú* (Rhizoma Atractylodis Macrocephalae) 12g, and *gān cǎo* (Radix et Rhizoma Glycyrrhizae) 6g.[2]

(3) Han Wu-xiang divides alopecia into three types:

1) Phlegm dampness with stasis heat

It should be treated by clearing heat, removing dampness, dispelling wind, removing phlegm, opening the channels, and relieving itching. The prescription is modified *Qū Fēng Huàn Jī Wán* (祛风换肌丸): *wēi líng xiān* (Radix et Rhizoma Clematidis) 10g, *shí chāng pú* (Rhizoma Acori Tatarinowii) 10g, *niú xī* (Radix Achyranthis Bidentatae) 10g, *cāng zhú* (Rhizoma Atractylodis) 10g, *tiān huā fěn* (Radix Trichosanthis) 10g, *chuān xiōng* (Rhizoma Chuanxiong) 10g, *dāng guī* (Radix Angelicae Sinensis) 10g, *hé shǒu wū* (Raw Radix Polygoni Multiflori) 30g, and *shēng gān cǎo* (Radix et Rhizoma Glycyrrhizae) 6g. Dosage is one bag per day. Drink warm, immediately after cooking.

2) Blood deficiency with wind dryness

It should be treated by nourishing blood and dispelling wind. The prescription is modified *Shén Yìng Yǎng Zhēn Dān* (神应养真丹): *chuān xiōng* (Rhizoma Chuanxiong), *dāng guī* (Radix Angelicae Sinensis), *bái sháo* (Radix Paeoniae Alba), *qiāng huó* (Rhizoma et Radix Notopterygii), *mù guā* (Fructus Chaenomelis), *tù sī zǐ* (Semen Cuscutae) 10g respectively, *tiān má* (Rhizoma Gastrodiae) 12g, and *zhì hé shǒu wū* (Radix Polygoni Multiflori Praeparata cum Succo Glycines Sotae) 30g. Dosage is one bag per day. Drink warm, immediately after cooking.

3) Liver and kidney deficiency

It should be treated by tonifying the liver and kidney, nourishing hair and helping hair to regrow. The prescription is modified *Qī Bǎo Měi Rán Dān* (七宝美髯丹): *zhì hé shǒu wū* (Radix Polygoni Multiflori

Praeparata cum Succo Glycines Sotae) 15g, *huái niú xī* (Radix Achyranthis Bidentatae) 10g, *bǔ gǔ zhī* (Fructus Psoraleae) 10g, *fú líng* (Poria) 10g, *tù sī zǐ* (Semen Cuscutae) 10g, *dāng guī* (Radix Angelicae Sinensis) 10g, and *gǒu qǐ zǐ* (Fructus Lycii) 10g. Dosage is one bag per day. Drink warm, immediately after cooking.[3]

(4) Yan Su-yun divided alopecia into two types:

1) Dampness accumulation due to spleen deficiency

This pattern usually occurs with oily types of androgenetic alopecia. The prescription is *Shēng Fà I Hào* (生发 I 号): *fú líng* (Poria) (with peel), *guì zhī* (Ramulus Cinnamomi), *bái zhú* (Rhizoma Atractylodis Macrocephalae), *zhì hé shǒu wū* (Radix Polygoni Multiflori Praeparata cum Succo Glycines Sotae), *bái xiān pí* (Cortex Dictamni), *kǔ shēn* (Radix Sophorae Flavescentis), *lù lù tōng* (Fructus Liquidambaris), and *gān cǎo* (Radix et Rhizoma Glycyrrhizae).

2) Kidney deficiency with blood dryness

This type of pattern usually occurs with dry androgenic alopecia. The prescription is *Shēng Fà II Hào* (生发 II 号): *dāng guī* (Radix Angelicae Sinensis), *shēng dì huáng* (Radix Rehmanniae), *gǒu qǐ zǐ* (Fructus Lycii), *sāng shèn* (Fructus Mori), *fú líng* (Poria), *chuān xiōng* (Rhizoma Chuanxiong), *bǎi zǐ rén* (Semen Platycladi), *zhì hé shǒu wū* (Radix Polygoni Multiflori Praeparata cum Succo Glycines Sotae), *lù lù tōng* (Fructus Liquidambaris), and *gān cǎo* (Radix et Rhizoma Glycyrrhizae).[4]

(5) Meng Ling-jun divided alopecia into four types:

Liver qi stagnation types are treated by coursing liver, regulating qi, and invigorating blood by using modified *Chái Hú Shū Gān Sǎn* (柴胡疏肝散).

Liver fire excess types are first treated by clearing liver fire, and then harmonizing and nourishing the blood with modified *Lóng Dǎn Xiè*

Gān Tāng (龙胆泻肝汤). Then use sour and sweet herbal medicines to generate blood and tonify liver by using modified *Sì Wù Tāng* (四物汤) and herbs that course the liver.

Damp-heat liver types can be treated by clearing damp-heat from liver with modified *Lóng Dǎn Xiè Gān Tāng*.

Liver blood deficiency types can be treated by nourishing blood and tonifying the liver with modified *Bǔ Gān Tāng* (补肝汤).[5]

(6) Wei Yue-gang divided alopecia into three types:

1) Damp-heat accumulation: It should be treated by clearing heat and removing dampness. The prescription is modified *Lóng Dǎn Xiè Gān Tāng* (龙胆泻肝汤): *lóng dǎn cǎo* (Radix et Rhizoma Gentianae) 5g, *huáng qín* (Radix Scutellariae) 10g, *shān zhī zǐ* (Fructus Gardeniae) 10g, *zé xiè* (Rhizoma Alismatis) 10g, *fú líng* (Poria) 10g, *dà huáng* (Raw Radix et Rhizoma Rhei) (decoct later) 5g, *chē qián zǐ* (Semen Plantaginis) (in bag) 10g, *mù tōng* (Caulis Akebiae) 5g, *cè bǎi yè* (Cacumen Platycladi) 15g, and *Liù Yī Sǎn* (六一散) (in bag) 10g.

2) Blood deficiency and wind dryness: It should be treated by nourishing blood and dispelling wind. The prescription is modified *Qū Fēng Huàn Jī Wán* (祛风换肌丸): *dāng guī* (Radix Angelicae Sinensis) 15g, *hé shǒu wū* (Raw Radix Polygoni Multiflori) 15g, *chuān xiōng* (Rhizoma Chuanxiong) 10g, *dān shēn* (Radix et Rhizoma Salviae Miltiorrhizae) 15g, *dà hú má* (Semen Sesami Nigrum) 10g, *jī xuè téng* (Caulis Spatholobi) 15g, *cāng zhú* (Rhizoma Atractylodis) 10g, *bái jí lí* (Fructus Tribuli) 10g, and *zhì gān cǎo* (Radix et Rhizoma Glycyrrhizae Praeparata cum Melle) 5g.

3) Liver and kidney deficiency: It should be treated by tonifying the liver and kidney. The prescription is modified *Liù Wèi Dì Huáng Wán* (六味地黄丸): *shēng dì huáng* (Radix Rehmanniae) 15g, *shú dì huáng* (Radix Rehmanniae Praeparata) 15g, *huái shān yào* (Rhizoma Dioscoreae) 15g, *shān zhū yú* (Fructus Corni) 10g, *zé xiè* (Rhizoma Alismatis) 10g, *fú líng*

(Poria) 10g, *hàn lián cǎo* (Herba Ecliptae) 15g, *nǚ zhēn zǐ* (Fructus Ligustri Lucidi) 15g, *hé shǒu wū* (Radix Polygoni Multiflori) 15g, *dān shēn* (Radix et Rhizoma Salviae Miltiorrhizae) 15g, and *zhì gān cǎo* (Radix et Rhizoma Glycyrrhizae Praeparata cum Melle) 5g. Decoct one bag of medicine per day.

If the patient feels dizzy, add *gōu téng* (Ramulus Uncariae Cum Uncis) and *tiān má* (Rhizoma Gastrodiae). If the patient has insomnia, add *yè jiāo téng* (Caulis Polygoni Multiflori) and *suān zǎo rén* (Semen Ziziphi Spinosae). If the patients have pain on the scalp, add *mù guā* (Fructus Chaenomelis) and *táo rén* (Semen Persicae).[6]

2. Specific Formulas

(1) *Shēng Fà Tāng* (生发汤)

The ingredients are: *shú dì huáng* (Radix Rehmanniae Praeparata), *gǒu qǐ zǐ* (Fructus Lycii), *huáng qí* (Radix Astragali), *dǎng shēn* (Radix Codonopsis), *fú líng* (Poria), *bái zhú* (Rhizoma Atractylodis Macrocephalae), *dān shēn* (Radix et Rhizoma Salviae Miltiorrhizae), *yì mǔ cǎo* (Herba Leonuri), *bái huā shé shé cǎo* (Herba Hedyotis Diffusae), *shān zhā* (raw Fructus Crataegi), and *shēng gān cǎo* (Radix et Rhizoma Glycyrrhizae). Decoct and take it twice a day for three months. If the hair is greasy with itching on the scalp, add *bái xiān pí* (Cortex Dictamni), *hǔ zhàng* (Rhizoma et Radix Polygoni Cuspidati), and *jīn qián cǎo* (Herba Lysimachiae). If there is dizziness and blurred vision, add *Qǐ Jiú Dì Huáng Wán* (杞菊地黄丸). If there is poor appetite, add *Xiāng Shā Liù Jūn Zǐ Tāng* (香砂六君子汤). If there is constipation, add *Qīng Jiě Piàn* (清解片): *dà huáng* (Radix et Rhizoma Rhei), *huáng qín* (Radix Scutellariae), *huáng bǎi* (Cortex Phellodendri Chinensis), and *cāng zhú* (Rhizoma Atractylodis). If there is back pain, irregular periods, disharmony in the *chong* and *ren* channels, add modified *Èr Xiān Tāng* (二仙汤).

96 cases of alopecia were treated with a rate of effectiveness of 91.67%.[7]

(2) *Zī Fàng Tāng* (滋发汤)

The ingredients are: *jí lí* (Fructus Tribuli) 15g, *shēng dì huáng* (Radix Rehmanniae) 15g, *bái xiān pí* (Cortex Dictamni) 15g, *dì fū zǐ* (Fructus Kochiae) 15g, *yě jú huā* (Flos Chrysanthemi Indici) 15g, *hēi zhī ma* (Semen Sesami Nigrum) 15g, *hé shǒu wū* (Radix Polygoni Multiflori) 15g, *mǔ dān pí* (Cortex Moutan) 12g, *chì sháo* (Radix Paeoniae Rubra) 12g, and *bái sháo* (Radix Paeoniae Alba) 12g.

Of the 72 cases treated, 23 were cured, 43 improved, and 6 cases had no effect. The rate of effectiveness was 91.7%.[8]

(3) *Cháng Qīng Fāng* (常青方)

The ingredients are: *hé shǒu wū* (Radix Polygoni Multiflori) 20g, *gě gēn* (Radix Puerariae Lobatae) 12g, *shēng dì huáng* (Radix Rehmanniae) 10g, *chán tuì* (Periostracum Cicadae) 10g, *xīn yí huā* (Flos Magnoliae) 10g, *dāng guī* (Radix Angelicae Sinensis) 10g, *yín yáng huò* (Herba Epimedii) 10g, *zǐ cǎo* (Radix Arnebiae) 10g, and *tù sī zǐ* (Semen Cuscutae) 10g. Blend the herbs into syrup, and take 50 ml three times a day.

Of the 39 cases, the rate of effectiveness was 100%.[9]

(4) *Qù Zhī Chōng Jì* (去脂冲剂)

The ingredients are: *mù guā* (Fructus Chaenomelis), *sāng bái pí* (Cortex Mori), *huáng qín* (Radix Scutellariae), *huáng bǎi* (Cortex Phellodendri Chinensis), *shān zhū yú* (Fructus Corni), *yù zhú* (Rhizoma Polygonati Odorati), and *shān zhā* (Fructus Crataegi). This formula was used to treat 110 cases.

The rate of effectiveness was 84.5%.[10]

(5) *Máo Fà Chōng Jì* (毛发冲剂)

The ingredients are: *shú dì huáng* (Radix Rehmanniae Praeparata), *dāng guī* (Radix Angelicae Sinensis), *nǚ zhēn zǐ* (Fructus Ligustri Lucidi), *qiāng huó* (Rhizoma et Radix Notopterygii), *hé shǒu wū* (Radix Polygoni Multiflori), *tiān má* (Rhizoma Gastrodiae), *mù guā* (Fructus Chaenomelis), *hóng huā* (Flos Carthami), *shān zhū yú* (Fructus Corni), *wǔ wèi zǐ* (Fructus Schisandrae Chinensis), *bái zhú* (Rhizoma Atractylodis Macrocephalae), *fú líng* (Poria), and *shēng gān cǎo* (Radix et Rhizoma Glycyrrhizae).

Of the 9 alopecia patients treated with this formula, there was an obvious effect in 4 cases, moderate effects in 4 cases, and no effect at all for 1 case.[11]

(6) *Jié Fū Yǐn* (洁肤饮)

The ingredients are: *sāng shèn* (Fructus Mori), *nǚ zhēn zǐ* (Fructus Ligustri Lucidi), *tù sī zǐ* (Semen Cuscutae), *hàn lián cǎo* (Herba Ecliptae), *bái huā shé shé cǎo* (Herba Hedyotis Diffusae), and *shān zhā* (Fructus Crataegi).

Of the 85 cases treated, 8 were cured, 37 showed an obvious effect, and 17 with no effect.[12]

(7) *Shēng Fà Wán* (生发丸)

The ingredients are: *dù zhòng* (Cortex Eucommiae) 100g, *gǒu qǐ zǐ* (Fructus Lycii) 100g, *bái kòu rén* (Fructus Amomi Kravanh) 100g, *nǚ zhēn zǐ* (Fructus Ligustri Lucidi) 15g, *dāng guī* (Radix Angelicae Sinensis) 150g, and *cè bǎi yè* (Cacumen Platycladi) 300g. The herbs were made into pills. The experimental group (70 patients) was treated with this formula while the control group of 65 patients were treated with vitamin B_1, vitamin B_6, oryzanal, cystinic acid, and levaminsole.

The experimental group results showed 45 cases cured, 21 improved, and 4 with no effect. The total rate of effectiveness 83.07%.[13]

(8) *Qū Shī Jiàn Fà Tāng* (祛湿健发汤)

The ingredients are: *bái zhú* (Rhizoma Atractylodis Macrocephalae)

15g, *zé xiè* (Rhizoma Alismatis) 10g, *fú líng* (Poria) 15g, *bì xiè* (Rhizoma Dioscoreae Hypoglaucae) 15g, *chē qián zǐ* (Semen Plantaginis) 10g, *sāng shèn* (Fructus Mori) 10g, *shēng dì huáng* (Radix Rehmanniae) 12g, *shú dì huáng* (Radix Rehmanniae Praeparata) 12g, *hé shǒu wū* (Radix Polygoni Multiflori) 15g, *bái xiān pí* (Cortex Dictamni) 15g, *chì shí zhī* (Halloysitum Rubrum) 12g, and *chuān xiōng* (Rhizoma Chuanxiong) 10g. Of the 9 cases treated, 3 were cured, 5 showed improvement, and 1 showed no effect.[14]

(9) *Chú Zhī Shēng Fà Tāng* (除脂生发汤)

The ingredients are: *fú líng* (Poria) 10g, *shān yào* (Rhizoma Dioscoreae) 15g, *yì yǐ rén* (Semen Coicis) 30g, *dān shēn* (Radix et Rhizoma Salviae Miltiorrhizae) 15g, *chì sháo* (Radix Paeoniae Rubra) 10g, *tiān má* (Rhizoma Gastrodiae) 10g, *gōu téng* (Ramulus Uncariae Cum Uncis) 10g, *yuǎn zhì* (Radix Polygalae) 10g, *nǚ zhēn zǐ* (Fructus Ligustri Lucidi) 15g, *hàn lián cǎo* (Herba Ecliptae) 15g, *tù sī zǐ* (Semen Cuscutae) 10g, *sāng shèn* (Fructus Mori) 30g. Decoct one bag of herbs per day and take it warm, twice a day.

Of the 34 cases, 3 were cured, 15 showed improvement, and 2 had showed effect. The total rate of effectiveness was 94.12%.[15]

(10) *Huó Xuè Shēng Fà Yǐn* (活血生发饮)

The ingredients are: *dāng guī* (Radix Angelicae Sinensis), *chuān xiōng* (Rhizoma Chuanxiong), *shēng dì huáng* (Radix Rehmanniae), *táo rén* (Semen Persicae), *hóng huā* (Flos Carthami), *bái sháo* (Radix Paeoniae Alba), *dān shēn* (Radix et Rhizoma Salviae Miltiorrhizae), *shān zhā* (Raw Fructus Crataegi), *sāng shèn* (Fructus Mori), *zé xiè* (Rhizoma Alismatis), *hé shǒu wū* (Radix Polygoni Multiflori), *chái hú* (Radix Bupleuri), *huáng qín* (Radix Scutellariae), and *dà zǎo* (Fructus Jujubae). Take one dose per day, twice a day. A half-month constituted one course of treatment.

If the patient has soreness and weakness in lower back and knees, red tongue, scanty coating, which is associated with kidney yin deficiency, add *hàn lián cǎo* (Herba Ecliptae) and *nǚ zhēn zǐ* (Fructus Ligustri Lucidi). If the patient has an itchy scalp and profuse dandruff, add *bái xiān pí* (Cortex Dictamni), *chán yī* (Periostracum Cicadae), and *bái jí lí* (Fructus Tribuli). If the patient has insomnia and excessive dreams, add *suān zǎo rén* (Semen Ziziphi Spinosae), *lóng gǔ* (Os Draconis), and *yè jiāo téng* (Caulis Polygoni Multiflori).

Of the 60 cases treated with this formula, 19 showed an obvious effect, 9 showed improvement, and 2 with no effect. The total rate of effectiveness was 93%.[16]

3. Acupuncture and Moxibustion

Li Lian-sheng used various acupuncture methods to treat alopecia.

(1) Filiform needle treatment

【Main points】 GB 20, DU 20, and EX-HN1.

【Point combination】

For excessive heat in stomach and intestines, add SP 10, ST 36, and BL 25.

For excessive heat in qi and blood, add DU 14 and BL 17.

For qi stagnation and blood stasis, add SP 6, BL 17, and needle PC 6 through to SJ 5.

For liver and kidney yin deficiency, add BL 18, BL 23, and ST 36.

For severe itching, add DU 14.

For excessive sebum secretions, add DU 23.

【Manipulation】 For excessive syndromes, use the sedating rotation technique; for deficient syndromes, use the tonifying rotation technique. Utilize this method every day or every other day for 20-30 minutes per treatment. Ten treatments constitute one course of treatment.

(2) Dermal needle treatment

Use dermal needle tapping on the affected areas once per day or every other day. Tap lightly for mild syndromes, and strongly for severe conditions. Ten treatments constitute one course of treatment.

(3) Bleeding treatment

Use three-edged needles on DU 14 6-8 times. Use antiseptic precautions around the local area of DU 14 before needle insertion. After insertion, use cupping to draw out blood. This bleeding technique is mainly used for excess patterns, heat patterns and stasis patterns.

(4) *Tuina*

Use the right thumb and index finger to massage bilateral GB 20. The left hand remains on the patient's forehead until he or she begins slightly sweating. Treatment is done 1-2 times per day. Ten treatments constitute one course of treatment.[17]

Yin Zhao-min used the scalp tapping method. Use fingertips to tap on the specific acupoints on the head, particularly on DU 20 and DU 15, as well as the local areas of alopecia, and along the governing vessel. Applied to 50 patients, the results showed that it had significant effects on slight to medium cases of alopecia. He believes that this type of treatment regulates the qi at the local points, clears the channels, and stimulates the hair follicles from dormant to active stages.

Yu Bing-lan mainly chose DU 20, DU 23, ST 8, and EX-HN1, combined with BL 23, GB 25 (*jīng mén*), and KI 3. Additionally, he used three *shu* and *mu* points to regulate kidney qi, as well as LU 9 (*tài yuān*) and KI 3 to clear the channels.

If there is insomnia, excessive dreams, add GB 20 and SP 6. If there is palpitation and stuffy chest, add HT 7 and PC 6. Utilize this treatment daily and retain the needles for half an hour.[19]

Yang Wei-qun used plum-blossom needles and regular needles for 12 cases of alopecia. For scalp acupuncture he used GB 20, ST 8, DU 23 and DU 20. For body acupuncture he used SP 6 and SP 10. After the acupuncture treatment, he used a plum-blossom needle to tap along the neck towards the forehead, *du* channel, and the three foot *yang* channels until the areas became red or slightly bleeding. This method should be used daily. Fifteen days constituted one course of treatment.

Of the 12 cases treated, 10 were cured, and 2 had obvious improvement.[20]

Mo Bing-seng treated alopecia using DU 20, GB 20, DU 23, ST 36, ST 44, and LV 3. In addition, he combined body acupuncture with ear acupuncture on CO14, CO18, CO13, AT4, and CO10. The rate of effectiveness was 95.12%.[21]

Xiang Yi gave treatments based on pattern differentiation.

Damp-heat pattern: Plum-blossom needle tapping along the *yangming* channel, and acupuncture on ST 36 and SP 6. Once the sebum secretion has decreased, rub ginger on the scalp to invigorate blood to rise up to the scalp to nourish the hair. If there is blood deficiency and wind dryness with liver and kidney deficiency, also add acupuncture on GB 20, DU 20, and ST 8.

For the 47 cases treated, the rate of effectiveness was 87%.[22]

Cheng Yi-wei used a plum-blossom to tap along the kidney and urinary bladder channels on the head, and along the gall bladder and urinary bladder channels on the back. Fifty-six cases were treated with plum-blossom tapping combined with a liquid mixture using *zào jiǎo cì* (Spina Gleditsiae) and *cè bǎi yè* (Cacumen Platycladi).

The rate of effectiveness was 98.1%.[23]

Experimental Studies

1. Research on the Efficacy of Single Chinese Medicinals

Jiubao Daode in Japan reported the effects of *hǎi jīn shā* (Spora Lygodii) on hair growth. He performed 5 experiments with rat models:

(1) Cultivating hair follicles on the upper lips of mice in order to

study the process of hair growth, he applied extract SL-ext for 48 hours, made from soaking *hǎi jīn shā* (Spora Lygodii) into 50% ethyl alcohol for 48 hours. It showed 15% hair growth.

(2) He also found that 2% or 4% SL-ext solution (varying with dosage) improved hair growth in these C3H mice. The strength is similar to 1% loniten.

(3) In vitro experiments showed that the extract SL-ext could inhibit 5α-reductase which would activate testosterone to transform into dihydrotestosterone.

(4) SL-ext improved hair growth on the backs of C 57 black mice.

(5) Exams found that the roots and spores of *hǎi jīn shā* (Spora Lygodii) also promoted hair growth.[24]

Japanese scholars cultivated hair follicles in mice and found that *huáng jīng* (Rhizoma Polygonati), *gōu téng* (Ramulus Uncariae Cum Uncis), and *sōng zǐ* can improve the DNA synthesis of hair follicles of mice depending on the concentration of the herbs. *Cì wǔ jiā* (Radix et Rhizoma seu Caulis Acanthopanacis Senticosi), *shuǐ fēi zhì* (Silybum marianum), and *sǎn mò huā yè* could also improve the hair growth with moderate consistency. Clinical studies have suggested good results for male alopecia.[26]

Inaoka conducted scientific research on the extracts of 80 herbal medicines and their effects on hair growth in mice. Eighteen of these 80 herbs could improve hair growth. The herbs found with significant effects were extracts from *shān zhā* (Fructus Crataegi), *nǚ zhēn zǐ* (Fructus Ligustri Lucidi), *zhū líng* (Polyporus), *bái jí* (Rhizoma Bletillae), and *jiè zǐ* (Semen Sinapis). Fatty acids are considered to be the main active ingredient in all these herbs.

Some other 16 herbal medicine extracts could inhibit hair growth including *qǐng má* (Abutili Theophrasti Herba seu Folium), *shēng jiāng* (Rhizoma Zingiberis Recens), *dà huáng* (Radix et Rhizoma Rhei), *rǔ xiāng*

(Olibanum), and *huò xiāng* (Herba Agastachis).[27]

Fan Wei-xin, Zhu Wen-yuan used the mice cirrus hair follicle external cultivation model, RT-PCR and gel density to conduct experimental research on *nǚ zhēn zǐ* (Fructus Ligustri Lucidi), *huáng qí* (Radix Astragali), and *bái zhǐ* (Radix Angelicae Dahuricae). The study suggested that *huáng qí* (Radix Astragali) could improve cirrus hair follicles growth in mice, though the mechanism is not clear. The main ingredient, oleanolic acid, from *nǚ zhēn zǐ* (Fructus Ligustri Lucidi) can improve externally cultivated hair follicles.[28] Later, through the research on 3H-TdR and the cultivation of morphology and the hair follicle growth rates, he conducted in-depth research comparing a formula decoction of 55 herbs to one single herb. He found that *nǚ zhēn zǐ* (Fructus Ligustri Lucidi), *bái zhǐ* (Radix Angelicae Dahuricae), *bái jí* (Rhizoma Bletillae), *jīng jiè* (Herba Schizonepetae), *huáng qí* (Radix Astragali), *bái jí lí* (Fructus Tribuli), and *gān cǎo* (Radix et Rhizoma Glycyrrhizae) can improve the hair growth on externally cultivated mice cirrus hair follicles. The main ingredient, oleanolic acid, in *nǚ zhēn zǐ* (Fructus Ligustri Lucidi) can improve hair growth, depending on its concentration. However, he found that *bǔ gǔ zhī* (Fructus Psoraleae), *bái liǎn* (Radix Ampelopsis), *fáng fēng* (Radix Saposhnikoviae), *dà huáng* (Radix et Rhizoma Rhei), *bīng láng* (Semen Arecae), and *qiàn cǎo* (Radix et Rhizoma Rubiae) significantly inhibited the growth of externally cultivated hair follicles.[29]

2. Research on the Efficacy of Herbal Prescriptions

Xuan Guo-wei treated 576 cases with by Chinese herbal medicine, *Yì Fà* Prescription. Of the 573 patients, 335 cases were cured (58.2%), 144 had significant improvements (25%), 83 had moderate effects. The total rate of effectiveness was 97.6%.

Patients were assigned into one of two groups: the herbal medicine group and the western medicine group. The herbal medicine group had better results than the control group ($p<0.01$). After treatment, hair loss, itching, and oiliness decreased. The external medicine was so gentle that the skin did not have any allergic reactions or side effects. Previous to treatment, there were no statistical differences between the two groups ($p>0.05$). After treatment, the two groups showed significant differences ($p<0.001$). The herbal treatment group's score was lower than the comparison group. The results from blood serum orchidic hormone (T), estradiol (E_2) showed that the average level of patients' blood T level was in the normal range. However it was higher than the healthy comparison group. After the treatment, the patients' blood T level lowered ($p<0.01$), and the E_2/T values increased. The results suggested that the treatment can reduce the abnormal blood T levels of alopecia patients and regulate E_2/T levels in order to normalize the endocrine system. Hair microscopy showed the effects of before and after treatment for alopecia. During alopecia, the hair analysis indicated that the microstructure of the hair shaft changed, superficial hair cells fell off, hair eroded, crusted, and ruptured, as reflected in a pathological state. The images of the newly grown hairs are similar to newly grown hairs of people without alopecia. Experimental research has shown that *Yì Fà* B external liniment can expand rabbit superficial dermis vasculature, increase blood flow volume, improve local microcirculation, improve hair follicle nutrients, and stimulate hair growth and regeneration. The microscopy found that the liniment can generate new hair follicles on the superficial dermis. On guinea pigs, it stopped itching on the local areas caused by histamine.[30] Chen Da-can observed the effect of this medicine for alopecia. He discovered that the Chinese Medicine *Yì Fà* Prescription was able to improve the immunity of the patients.[31]

Liu Wei studied the effects of the Chinese medicine, *Yì Fà* Formula, for treating androgenetic alopecia. The herbs in the formula are *nǚ zhēn zǐ* (Fructus Ligustri Lucidi) 20g, *tù sī zǐ* (Semen Cuscutae) 20g, *huáng qí* (Radix Astragali) 15g, *hé shǒu wū* (Radix Polygoni Multiflori) 15g, *pú gōng yīng* (Herba Taraxaci) 15g, *dān shēn* (Radix et Rhizoma Salviae Miltiorrhizae) 15g, and *gān cǎo* (Radix et Rhizoma Glycyrrhizae) 10g. He researched its effects on hair follicle vascular endothelial cell growth factor (VEGF) mRNA in cultured human scalp hair follicles. The result indicated that 10% and 20% Chinese medicine with medical serum VEGF mRNA is significantly better than 10% empty blood serum group ($p<0.01$). It showed that the *Yì Fà* formula can stimulate the hair papillae cells to secrete VEGF, and promote the expression of VEGF mRNA on hair cultured hair follicles.[32]

Zhao Dang-sheng studied androgenetic alopecia by investigating the effects of testosterone injections at the neck of mice. At the same time, he gave intragastric administration in high, medium and low doses of *Zhi Tuo Ling*.

The ingredients of *Zhi Tuo Ling*: *dān shēn* (Radix et Rhizoma Salviae Miltiorrhizae) *hé shǒu wū* (Radix Polygoni Multiflori), *shān zhā* (Fructus Crataegi), *rén shēn yè* (Folium Ginseng), *shēng dì huáng* (Radix Rehmanniae), *dà huáng* (Radix et Rhizoma Rhei), *pú gōng yīng* (Herba Taraxaci), *huáng jīng* (Rhizoma Polygonati), *dāng guī* (Radix Angelicae Sinensis), and *gān cǎo* (Radix et Rhizoma Glycyrrhizae).

He made observations of depilation in the alopecia regions, analyzed the blood for 60 days, and detected both group's levels of serum andrusol (T), destradiol (E_2) and T/E_2 by radio-immunity treatment. Compared to the comparison groups, the mice in the experimental group showed increased serum T and T/E_2 levels. The quantity of depilation in alopecia regions increased significantly ($p<0.01$). The mice in the other group displayed decreased serum T and T/E_2 levels, and the quantity of depilation also decreased ($p<0.01$ or $p<0.05$). Results suggest that androgenetic alopecia mice have significant levels of irregular hormone activity (especially androgen). Furthermore, *Zhi Tuo Ling* can regulate

T/E$_2$ levels back to normal as a way to prevent alopecia.[33]

3. Syndrome Differentiation Studies

Chen Xiu-yang researched the relationship among androgen receptor expression, the distribution regularity in the local area of the androgenetic alopecia and Chinese medicine syndromes. He divided 80 androgenetic alopecia patients into two groups: (1) Damp-heat of the spleen and stomach and (2) Deficiency of the liver and kidney. He used immunohistochemical methods to compare the androgen receptor levels in alopecia regions on the scalp compared to regions without signs of alopecia. He found that in the damp-heat in stomach and spleen group, sebaceous follicles in the alopecia regions increased in size and volume. The percentage of androgen receptor cells in the sweat glands and sebaceous follicles was significantly higher in this group than the deficiency in liver and kidney group ($p<0.05$). However, the androgen receptor levels on the epidermis, root sheath, and hair papilla in these two groups were not statistically significant ($p>0.05$). This research suggests that the pathological characteristics and the quantity of androgen receptors in alopecia regions are closely related to Chinese medicine syndrome differentiation for androgenetic alopecia. This provides a new perspective for discussing the mechanism of Chinese medicine in regulating the endocrine system.[34]

REFERENCES

[1] Zhu Ren-kang. Pattern Differentiation Of Alopecia (脱发证治). *Journal of Traditional Chinese Medicine* (中医杂志). 1986, 27 (12) :10

[2] Ta Guo-wei, Fan Rui-qiang. *Chinese Medicine Treatment on Dermatosis and Venereal Disease* (皮肤性病中医治疗全书). Guang Zhou: Guangdong Science and Technology Publishing House, 1996.321

[3] Han Wu-xiang, Ye Qian-yi. Syndrome Differentiation Treatment of 290 Seborrheic Alopecia Patients (辨证治疗脂溢性脱发290例). *Zhejiang Journal of Traditional Chinese Medicine* (浙江中医杂志). 1996, (6): 258

[4] Yan Su-yuan. Clinical Experience of Chinese Medicine Treating 764 Alopecia Cases (中药治疗脱发证764例临床小结). *New Journal of Traditional Chinese Medicine* (新中医). 1988, 20 (10): 35

[5] Meng Ling-jun. The Mechanism of Liver Syndrome Differentiation on Alopecia (脱发从肝论治的机理). *Jiangsu Journal of Traditional Chinese Medicine* (江苏中医). 1999, 20(3): 7

[6] Wei Yue-gang. Syndrome Differentiation on Treating 84 Seborrheic Alopecia Patients (辨证治疗脂溢性脱发84例). *Journal of Nanjing University of Traditional Chinese Medicine University:·Natural Science* (南京中医药大学学报·自然科学版). 2002,18(4): 251

[7] Meng Xin. Sheng Fa Tang Treating 90 Seborrheic Alopecia Cases (生发汤治疗脂溢性脱发90例). *Liaoning Journal of Traditional Chinese Medicine* (辽宁中医杂志). 1994, (7) :319

[8] Tan Rong-ju. The Effects of Zi Fa Tang In Treating 72 Seborrheic Alopecia Cases(滋发汤治疗脂溢性脱发72例疗效观察). *Shanxi Journal of Traditional Chinese Medicine* (陕西中医). 1987, 8 (2): 59

[9] Zhu Dao-ben. Sixty Cases of Chang Qing Fang Treating Seborrheic Alopecia and Alopecia Areata (常青方治疗脂溢性脱发和斑秃60例). *Hubei Journal of Traditional Chinese medicine* (湖北中医杂志). 1985, (3): 27

[10] Xiang Xi-rei. Qu Zhi Chong Ji in Treating 110 Cases of Seborrheic Alopecia (去脂冲剂治疗脂溢性脱发110例). *Chinese Journal of Integrated Traditional and Western Medicine* (中西医结合杂志). 1990, 10 (4): 244

[11] Liang Jian, Liu Shi-ming, Ding Su-xian. Twenty-three Cases of Mao Fa Chong Ji Treating Alopecia (毛发冲剂治疗脱发23例报告). *Tianjin Journal of Traditional Chinese Medicine* (天津中医). 1990, (3): 16

[12] Yan Pei-jun. Research on Zi Yi Jie Fu Yin Treating Seborrheic Alopecia and Domdo (自拟洁肤饮治疗脂溢性脱发和痤疮疗效观察). *Shanghai Journal of Traditional Chinese Medicine* (上海中医药杂志). 1995, (9): 38

[13] Xing Yue-er. Seventy Cases of Sheng Fa Wan In Treating Alopecia (生发丸治疗脱发)70例. *Chinese Journal of Medical Aesthetics and Cosmetology* (中国医学美学美容杂志). 1994, 2(3): 137

[14] Chen Qi-xiong. Nine Cases of Qu Shi Jian Fa Tang Treating Seborrheic Alopecia (祛湿健发汤治疗脂溢性脱发9例). *Guangxi Journal of Traditional Chinese Medicine* (广西中医药). 2000, 23(1): 49

[15] Chen Wei. Thirty-four Cases of Chu Zhi Sheng Fa Tang and External Treatment Treating Seborrheic Alopecia (除脂生发汤配外治法治疗脂溢性脱发34例). *Hebei Journal of Traditional Chinese Medicine* (河北中医). 2005, 27(2): 101-102

[16] Fang Yu-lian, Xu Yan-ping. Sixty Cases Clinical Research of Huo Xue Sheng Fa Yin Treating Seborrheic Alopecia (活血生发饮治疗脂溢性脱发60例临床观察). *Chinese Journal of Traditional Medical Science and Technology* (中国中医药科技). 2005，l2(4): 215

[17] Li Lian-sheng. Acupuncture Treatment for Dermatopathy (皮肤病针灸疗法). Tianjin: Tianjin Science and Technology Publishing House, 1993.370

[18] Yin Zhao-min. Clinical Research of Using The Scalp Plum Blossom Tapping Treatment Treating Alopecia Premature on 50 Cases (头皮叩击治疗早秃50例临床观察). *Shanxi Journal of Traditional Chinese Medicine* (山西中医). 1993, 9(5): 32

[19] Yu Bing-lan, Yu Ming-lan, Zhang Li Juan. Acupuncture Treatment for Alopecia (脱发的针刺治疗). *Journal of Clinical Acupuncture and Moxibustion* (针灸临床杂志). 1997, 13(2): 40-41

[20] Yang Wei-qun. Twelve Clinical Case Studies of Using Acupuncture and Plum-Blossom Technique In Treating Seborrheic Alopecia (针刺配合梅花针治疗脂溢性脱发12例疗效观察). *Journal of Clinical Acupuncture and Moxibustion* (针灸临床杂志). 1997, 13(2):11

[21] Mo Bing-seng. Clinical Research of A Combined Treatment for Seborrheic Alopecia(综合疗法治疗脂溢性脱发疗效观察). *Shanghai Journal of Acupuncture* (上海针灸杂志). 1999, 18(2):48

[22] Xiang Yi. Eighty-three Cases of Plum-Blossom Needle Technique For Seborrheic Alopecia (梅花针治疗脱发83例). *Journal of Nanjing University of Traditional Chinese Medicine University* (南京中医药大学学报). 1996, 12(2):51

[23] Cheng Yi-wei. Fifty-six Cases of Using Plum-Blossom Needle and Local Application Treating Seborrheic Alopecia (梅花针叩刺配合局部用药治疗脂溢性脱发56例疗效观察). *Journal of Tianjin College of Traditional Chinese Medicine* (天津中医学院学报). 1997, 16(8):16

[24] The Effects of *hǎi jīn shā* (Spora Lygodii) for hair growth (海金沙生发的效果). *Foreign Medical Sciences of Chinese Medicine* (国外医学中医中药分册). 2002, 24(4):246.

[25] Ji Bing Gui Yi Lang. Dried Medical herb's effect on Cultivating DNA Synthesis of Mice Hair Follicles (生药对培养小鼠毛囊DNA合成的影响). *Day Leather Institute Memory* (日皮会志). 1993, 103(3):368

[26] Sang Ming Long Yi Lang. The Animal Exam and The Effect of Growing Hair Using *Sāng Bái Pí* (Cortex Mori)'s extract (桑白皮浸出物的动物试验及临床生发效果). *West and Janpan Leather Surname* (西日皮唐). l996, 58(4):619

[27] Li Zong-you, Li Jing-chun. The Effects of Herb Extracts on Hair Growth and The Extracts of The Active Ingredient of *Zhū Líng* (Polyporus) (草药提取物对毛发生长的作用及猪苓中活性成分的分离). *Foreign Medical·Branch Volume of Chinese Medicine* (国外医学·中医中药分册). 1995, 17(2):17-18

[28] Fan Wei-xin, Zhu Wen-yuan. The Effects of *Nu Zhen Zi* on the Expression of mRNA Growth Factor during the Growth Period of Mice Hair Follicle (女贞子等中药对小鼠毛囊生长周期中生长因子mRNA表达的影响). *Chinese Journal of Dermatology* (中华皮肤科杂志). 2000, 33(4): 229-231

[29] Fan Wei-xin, Zhu Wen-yuan. The Research on Features of 55 Kinds of Herbs and Their Effects on Mice Barbel Hair Follicle External Cultivation Biology (55种中药对小鼠触须毛囊体外培养生物学特性的研究). *Journal of Clinical Dermatology* (临床皮肤科杂志). 2001, 30(2): 81-84

[30] Xuan Guo-Wei, Chen Da-can, Hu Dong-liu. The Clinical and Experimental Research of Chinese Medicine Yi Fa Treating Seborrheic Alopecia (中药益发治疗脂溢性脱发的临床与实验研究). *Journal of Practical Medicine* (实用医学杂志). 1997,13 (4): 265

[31] Chen Da-can, Xuan Guo-wei, Hu Dong-liu. The Research of 319 Cases Using Chinese Medicine Preparation, Yi Fa Treatment, on Alopecia Areata (中药制剂益发治疗斑秃319例临床疗效观察). *Journal of Guangzhou University of Traditional Chinese Medicine* (广州中医药大学学报). 1997,(3, 4):159

[32] Liu Wei, Chen Da-can, Han Ling. Chinese Medicine Yi Fa Formula's Effect on Externally Cultivating the Expression of the Human Hair Follicle VEGFmRNA (中药"益发"复方对体外培养人

毛囊VEGFmRNA表达的影响). *Chinese Journal of Current Practical Medicine* (中国现代实用医学杂志). 2005(4):1-3

[33] Zhao Dang-sheng, Li Shu-xia, Zhao Chun-lin. Zhi Tuo Ling's Regulation of Androgen in Mice and Its Influence on Hair Loss ("止脱灵"对实验性大鼠雄激素的调节及对毛发脱落的影响). *Journal of Gansu College of Traditional Chinese Medicine* (甘肃中医学院学报). 2005, 22(1):12-14

[34] Chen Xiu-yang, Chen Da-chan. The Discussion Of Pathological Characteristics andAndrogen Receptors on the Scalp of Androgenetic Alopecia Patients and Its Relation to Chinese Medicine Syndromes (雄激素性脱发患者受损头皮的病理特征及雄激素受体与中医证候关系的探讨). *Journal of Guangzhou University of Traditional Chinese Medicine* (广州中医药大学学报). 2004, 21(3):169

Index by Disease Names and Symptoms

A

accumulated heat in the lung and stomach, 029
acne, 005
acne associated with lung and stomach accumulated heat, 021
alopecia totalis, 075, 076
alopecia universalis, 075
anxiety, 075
atrophic scar, 024
aversion to cold, 078

B

blackhead, 027, 031
blood and essence deficiency, 098
blood deficiency, 132
blood deficiency and wind dryness, 192, 213
blood deficiency with wind dryness, 209, 211
blood heat, 039, 087
blood heat and wind dryness, 161, 162, 208, 210
blood heat engendering wind, 077
blood heat in the lung and stomach channels, 008
blood stasis, 029, 079, 087, 135
blurred vision, 084

C

chest and rib-side pain, 082
chest distress, 080
congealing yin cold, 188
constipation, 011, 097
cyst, 005, 030
cystic acne, 024

D

damp-heat, 163, 191, 192, 194, 196
damp-heat accumulating upwards, 209, 210
damp-heat accumulation, 213
damp-heat in the spleen and stomach, 161
dampness accumulation due to spleen deficiency, 212
dampness predominating over heat, 031
damp obstruction, 168
delayed menstruation, 026, 036
depressed internal fire, 105
disharmony of the penetrating and conception vessels, 008, 013, 036
distending pain in the breasts, 013
distending pain in the chest and hypochondria, 203
dizziness, 078, 084
dream-disturbed sleep, 009, 011
dry mouth, 162
dryness-heat, 031
dual deficiencies of qi and blood, 077
dusky purple tongue, 080

E

early menstruation, 014
exuberant lung-stomach heat, 011
exuberant wind, 168

F

fatigue, 197
five-center heat, 163
flaky alopecia, 082
fullness and oppression in the chest and abdomen, 105

G

ghost-licked head, 076, 131
ghost- shaved head, 076
ghost shaving head, 133
glossy scalp wind, 076, 133, 134

H

hair loss, 078
headache, 080
heat induced by blood deficiency, 086
heat predominating over dampness, 031
hyperactivity of fire due to yin deficiency, 029

I

infection, 114
insomnia, 075, 078, 080, 084, 088, 097, 101, 165, 196, 203
insufficiency of the liver and kidney, 077, 100
irregular menstruation, 013
irritability, 080, 097
itching, 088

K

kidney deficiency with blood dryness, 212
kidney yin deficiency, 007, 176

L

lethargy, 084
liver and kidney deficiency, 108, 165, 209, 210, 211, 213
liver and kidney yin deficiency, 105
liver constraint and blood deficiency, 181
liver constraint and qi stagnation, 015
liver constraint transforming into fire, 082
liver depression and blood stasis, 077
lung and stomach accumulated heat, 027
lung heat, 034, 042
lung qi deficiency, 177
lung wind, 028
lung wind acne, 006
lung yin deficiency, 177

N

nightmare, 080
nodule, 005, 022, 030

O

oily dandruff, 203

P

palpitation, 084
papule, 005, 025
pessimism, 095
phlegm and blood stasis binding together, 008
phlegm dampness with stasis heat, 211
phlegm stasis, 028
poor appetite, 088
poor memory, 165
postpartum hemorrhaging, 121
profuse dreaming, 196
pustule, 005, 022, 024, 027, 030

Q

qi and blood deficiency, 100
qi deficiency, 197
qi stagnation and blood stasis, 203

R

restlessness, 080, 097

S

scalp itchiness, 162
seborrheic dermatitis, 171
seminal emission, 078
somnolence, 084
soreness and weakness

of the lower back and
knees, 165
sorrow, 095
spleen-stomach
disharmony, 101
spleen deficiency leading
to damp encumbrance,
181
spontaneous sweating, 197
stabbing pain on the scalp,
080
stress, 095

T

thin falling hair, 163
thirst, 097
tinnitus, 078

V

vertigo, 078
vexation, 009

W

weak nutritive qi and
strong defensive qi, 190

whitehead, 031
wind dryness, 171
wind dryness due to
blood deficiency, 101
wind heat in the lung
channel, 042

Y

yang qi deficiency, 188
yin deficiency generating
internal heat, 009, 020
yin essence deficiency, 191,
198

Index by Chinese Medicinals and Formulas

A

Aloe, 043
Alumen, 048, 093, 171, 178
Alumen dehydratum, 193
Arillus Longan, 177
Armeniacae Semen Amarum, 177

B

bǎi bù, 063, 173
bái fán, 171
bái guǒ, 017
bái guǒ rén, 056
bǎi hé, 096, 177
bái huā shé shé cǎo, 018, 022, 026, 030
Bái Hǔ Tāng, 032
bái jiāng cán, 041
bái jiè zǐ, 189
bái jí lí, 064
bái sháo, 014, 081, 083, 104
bái xiān pí, 162, 164, 196
bái zhǐ, 052
bái zhú, 085, 101, 164, 179, 183, 184
bǎi zǐ rén, 176
bān máo, 093, 139, 142, 173
Bān Tū Wán, 086
bàn xià, 092
běi xìng rén, 020
biǎn dòu, 046
Bīng Fà Shēng Zhǎng Fāng, 172
bīng piàn, 048
bì xiè, 164, 179
Bombyx Batryticatus, 041, 196
Borneolum, 018
Borneolum Syntheticum, 048
Bǔ Gān Tāng, 213
bǔ gǔ zhī, 124
Bulbus Lilii, 096, 177

C

Cacumen Platycladi, 030, 050, 093, 096, 147, 171, 173, 193, 199, 202
Calamina, 018
Camellia sinensis O. Ktze, 030
cāng ěr zǐ, 171, 172, 178
cāng zhú, 057
Cannabis Folium, 172, 174, 200
cǎo wū, 141
Caulis Impatientis, 094, 171, 193
Caulis Polygoni Multiflori, 092, 104
Caulis Spatholobi, 109
cè bǎi yè, 030, 050, 093, 096, 147, 171, 173, 193, 199, 202
chái hú, 013, 014, 043, 081
Chái Hú Shū Gān Sǎn, 212
Chái Hú Shū Gān Tāng, 013
chán tuì, 027, 162
chǎo é zhú, 029
chǎo sān léng, 029
chá shù gēn, 030
chén pí, 082, 105
chē qián cǎo, 055
chē qián zǐ, 179, 183
chì sháo, 021, 024, 028, 029, 083
chì shí zhī, 179
chóng lóu, 063
chuān liàn zǐ, 203
chuān shān jiǎ, 012
chuān xiōng, 041, 081, 104, 183, 184

Chú Zhī Shēng Fà Tāng, 217
cí shí, 084
Colla Cornus Cervi, 134, 189
Concha Ostreae, 096, 196
Cordyceps, 093
Cornu Bubali, 043
Cornu Cervi, 189
Cortex Dictamni, 162, 164, 196
Cortex Eucommiae, 176
Cortex Lycii, 041
Cortex Mori, 021, 027, 040, 042, 094, 171
Cortex Moutan, 024, 028, 083, 106
Cuò Chuāng Gāo, 066
Cuò Chuāng Píng, 022, 040
Cuò Chuāng Qīng Xiāo Yǐn, 047
Cuò Chuāng Yǐn, 040
Cuò Líng Dīng, 016
Cuò Líng Shuāng, 016
Cuò Yù Sǎn, 050

D

dà huáng, 011, 174
dài zhě shí, 080, 174
dāng guī, 026, 081, 103, 104, 109, 123, 144, 162, 192
Dāng Guī Lú Huì Wán, 043
Dāng Guī Piàn, 087
dāng guī wěi, 050
dǎng shēn, 085
dān shēn, 010, 012, 026, 029, 030, 035, 197, 204
Dān Zhī Xiāo Yáo Sǎn, 032, 040
Dān Zhī Xiāo Yáo Wán, 015
dàn zhú yè, 043
dà qīng yè, 042
dà zǎo, 177
Dens Dragonis, 196
Diān Dǎo Sǎn, 055
dì fū zǐ, 030, 050, 196
dì gǔ pí, 041
dì huáng, 109
dì yú, 063
dōng chóng xià cǎo, 093
dōng qīng zǐ, 106
dù zhòng, 176

E

Èr Chén Tāng, 041
Èr Xiān Tāng, 032
Èr Zhì Wán, 035, 040, 083, 111, 168
é zhú, 064

F

fáng fēng, 056, 162
féi gān shí, 018
Fěn Cì Jiān, 047
Flos Albiziae, 143
Flos Carthami, 012, 029, 033, 081, 098, 103, 139, 173
Flos Celosiae Cristatae, 101
Flos Chrysanthemi, 027, 162
Flos Chrysanthemi Indici, 040, 171
Flos Genkwa, 113
Flos Lonicerae Japonicae, 040
Flos Rhododendri Mollis, 143
Flos Rosae Rugosae, 055
Folium Eriobotryae, 021, 027, 028, 040
Folium Isatidis, 042
Folium Mori, 019, 107, 172
Fructus Cannabis, 030
Fructus Chaenomelis, 099
Fructus Cnidii, 093
Fructus Corni, 124, 166
Fructus Crataegi, 013, 023, 026, 046, 201
Fructus Forsythiae, 040
Fructus Gardeniae, 029, 106
Fructus Hordei Germinatus, 205
Fructus Jujubae, 177
Fructus Kochiae, 030, 050, 196
Fructus Ligustri Lucidi, 010, 012, 014, 029, 041, 097, 100, 166, 183, 195
Fructus Liquidambaris, 180
Fructus Lycii, 079, 099, 100, 102, 111, 166

Fructus Mori, 083, 096, 099, 101, 107, 109, 176, 183
Fructus Psoraleae, 124
Fructus Rosae Laevigatae, 187
Fructus Rubi, 176
Fructus Schisandrae Chinensis, 101
Fructus Toosendan, 203
Fructus Tribuli, 064, 162
Fructus Trichosanthis, 065
Fructus Viticis, 187
Fructus Xanthii, 171, 172, 178
Fù Fāng Shé Cǎo Tāng, 065
fú líng, 079, 085, 164
Fú Líng Wán, 045
fù pén zǐ, 176

G

Galla Chinensis, 171
gān dì huáng, 176
gān shè xiāng, 051
gān sōng, 173
gān suì, 113
gǒu qǐ zǐ, 079, 099, 100, 102, 111, 166
guì zhī, 189
Guì Zhī Jiā Sháo Yào Tāng, 190
Gù Shèn Shēng Fà Tāng, 099
gǔ suì bǔ, 093, 140
Gypsum Fibrosum, 021, 027, 048

H

Haematitum, 080, 174
Hǎi Ài Tāng, 133
hǎi zǎo, 019, 024, 029, 204
Halloysitum Rubrum, 179
hàn lián cǎo, 010, 012, 014, 041, 091, 166
hé huān huā, 143
hēi dòu, 109
hēi zhī ma, 106, 111, 183
henry chloranthus, 093
Herba Artemisiae Scopariae, 022, 042, 164, 196
Herba Cistanches, 026
Herba Ecliptae, 010, 014, 041, 091, 139, 147, 166
Herba Epimedii, 026, 144, 189, 198
Herba Eupatorii, 192
Herba Hedyotis Diffusae, 018, 022, 026, 030, 196
Herba Houttuyniae, 012, 013
Herba Leonuri, 026, 064, 204
Herba Lophatheri, 043
Herba Plantaginis, 055
Herba Portulacae, 054
Herba Schizonepetae, 050, 056, 162
Herba Taraxaci, 012, 013, 024, 040, 064, 099
Herba Taxilli, 100, 176
Herba Violae, 027, 040, 063

hé shǒu wū, 092, 099, 103, 123, 176, 180
Hé Shǒu Wū Kǔ Shēn Hé Jì, 052
hé táo rén, 145, 176
hóng huā, 012, 029, 033, 081, 098, 103, 139, 173
huái niú xī, 124
huā jiāo, 131, 134, 140, 173
huáng dān, 018
huáng jīng, 109, 166
huáng lián, 174
Huáng Lián Jiě Dú Tāng, 040
huáng qí, 085, 102, 145, 192, 195, 197
Huáng Qí Jiàn Zhōng Tāng, 134
huáng qín, 021, 027, 174
Huà Yū Sàn Jié Wán, 028
huǒ má rén, 030
Huó Xuè Shēng Fà Yǐn, 217
hǔ zhàng, 022, 026, 030, 063

I

Ilicis Chinensis Semen, 106

J

jiāng cán, 196
Jiàn Pí Wán, 168
jiāo mù, 063
Jiā Wèi Sì Wù Tāng, 144
Jiā Wèi Xiāo Yáo Sǎn, 043

Jiě Dú Huà Yū Tāng, 053
Jié Fū Yǐn, 216
jī guān huā, 101
jí lí, 162
jīng jiè, 050, 056, 162
Jīn Huáng Gāo, 034
Jīn Huáng Sǎn, 050
Jīn Jú Xiāng Jiān Jì, 065
jīn sù lán, 093
jīn yīng zǐ, 187
jīn yín huā, 040
Jīn Yín Huā Tāng, 055
jī xuè téng, 109
jué míng zǐ, 144
jú huā, 027, 162
jú pí, 041

K

Kè Tū Níng Dīng, 147
kū fán, 048, 193
kūn bù, 019, 024, 029, 204
kǔ shēn, 030, 050, 162, 171, 178, 180

L

Lantana camara, 051
Liáng Xuè Xiāo Fēng Sǎn, 162
lián qiào, 040
Lián Shí Sǎn, 051
lián zǐ, 096, 177
líng líng xiāng, 173
liú huáng, 202
Liù Wèi Dì Huáng Wán, 168, 194
lóng chǐ, 196

lóng dǎn cǎo, 043
Lóng Dǎn Xiè Gān Tāng, 040
Lóng Dǎn Xiè Gān Wán, 168
lóng yǎn ròu, 177
lú huì, 043
lù jiǎo jiāo, 134, 189
lù jiǎo piàn, 189
lù lù tōng, 180

M

mǎ chǐ xiàn, 054
Magnetitum, 084
mài dōng, 023, 029
mài yá, 205
màn jīng zǐ, 187
Máo Fà Chōng Jì, 215
má yè, 172, 174, 200
méi guī huā, 055
Méi Huā Diǎn Shé Wán, 015
méi piàn, 018
míng fán, 093, 178
mò hàn lián, 139, 147
mǔ dān pí, 021, 024, 028, 083, 106
mù guā, 099
mǔ lì, 096, 196
Mylabris, 093, 139, 142, 173

N

nào yáng huā, 143
niú xī, 079
nǚ zhēn zǐ, 010, 012, 014, 029, 041, 097, 100, 166, 183, 195

P

paprika, 139
pèi lán, 192
Pericarpium Citri Reticulatae, 041, 082, 105
Pericarpium Zanthoxyli, 131, 134, 140, 173
Periostracum Cicadae, 027, 162
Píng Cuò Tāng, 023
Pí Pá Qīng Fèi Yǐn, 021, 028, 032, 040, 041, 042
pí pá yè, 021, 027, 028, 040
Pí Zhī Cā Jì, 172
Placenta Hominis, 198
Plumbum rubrum, 018
Polyporus, 179
Poria, 079, 085, 164
pú gōng yīng, 012, 013, 024, 040, 064, 099
Pǔ Jì Xiāo Dú Yǐn, 046

Q

qiāng huó, 111
Qī Bǎo Měi Rán Dān, 078, 086, 166
Qǐ Jú Dì Huáng Wán, 087
Qīng Fèi Qū Zhī Fāng, 066
Qīng Fèi Xiāo Dú Yǐn, 040
Qīng Rè Huà Yū Xiāo Chuāng Sǎn, 053
Qīng Wèi Sǎn, 044

Qīng Yíng Tāng, 043
quán guā lóu, 065
Qū Shī Jiàn Fà Tāng, 216
Qù Zhī Chōng Jì, 215
Qū Zhī Shēng Fà Dīng, 205

R

Radix Achyranthis Bidentatae, 079, 124
Radix Aconiti Kusnezoffii, 141
Radix Aconiti Lateralis Praeparata, 189
Radix Angelicae Dahuricae, 052, 173, 203
Radix Angelicae Sinensis, 026, 050, 081, 103, 104, 109, 123, 144, 162, 192
Radix Astragali, 085, 102, 145, 192, 195, 197
Radix Bupleuri, 013, 014, 043, 081
Radix Codonopsis, 085
Radix Curcumae, 012, 014, 143, 203
Radix et Rhizoma Nardostachyos, 173
Radix et Rhizoma Rhei, 011, 174
Radix et Rhizoma Salviae Miltiorrhizae, 010, 012, 026, 029, 030, 035, 197, 204
Radix et Rhizoma Sophorae Tonkinensis, 063
Radix Gentianae, 043
Radix Ginseng, 173
Radix Ipomoeae Cairicae, 109
Radix Kansui, 113
Radix Ophiopogonis, 023, 029
Radix Paeoniae Alba, 014, 081, 083, 104
Radix Paeoniae Rubra, 021, 024, 028, 029, 083
Radix Panacis Quinquefolii, 092
Radix Polygoni Multiflori, 092, 099, 103, 123, 176, 180
Radix Polygoni multiflori, 023, 026, 029
Radix Polygoni Multiflori Praeparata cum Succo Glycines Sotae, 079, 085, 147, 165, 166
Radix Pseudostellariae, 107, 110, 195
Radix Rehmanniae, 010, 012, 021, 023, 024, 026, 028, 029, 083, 106, 107, 109, 162, 176, 183
Radix Rehmanniae Praeparata, 099, 101, 102, 104, 106, 124, 134, 180
Radix Sanguisorbae, 063
Radix Saposhnikoviae, 056, 162
Radix Scrophulariae, 023, 026, 083, 107
Radix Scutellariae, 021, 027, 174
Radix Sophorae Flavescentis, 030, 050, 162, 178, 180
Radix Stemonae, 063, 173
Radix Trichosanthis, 023, 029
Ramulus Cinnamomi, 189
raw Fructus Crataegi, 030
rén shēn, 173
Rén Shēn Yǎng Róng Tāng, 085
Rén Shēn Yǎng Róng Wán, 086
Rhizoma Alismatis, 010, 164, 179, 183
Rhizoma Anemarrhenae, 010
Rhizoma Atractylodis, 057
Rhizoma Atractylodis Macrocephalae, 085, 101, 164, 179, 183, 184
Rhizoma Chuanxiong, 041, 081, 104, 183, 184
Rhizoma Cimicifugae, 044
Rhizoma Coptidis, 174
Rhizoma Curculiginis, 198
Rhizoma Curcumae, 029, 064
Rhizoma Cyperi, 041, 082, 143
Rhizoma Dioscoreae Hypoglaucae, 164, 179

Rhizoma Drynariae, 093, 140
Rhizoma et Radix Notopterygii, 111
Rhizoma Gastrodiae, 142
Rhizoma Kaempferiae, 093
Rhizoma Paridis, 024, 063
Rhizoma Pinelliae, 092
Rhizoma Polygonati, 109, 166
Rhizoma Polygoni Cuspidati, 022, 026, 030, 063
Rhizoma Smilacis Glabrae, 011, 101, 196
Rhizoma Sparganii, 029, 030
Rhizoma Zingiberis Recens, 091, 117, 131, 147, 173
ròu cōng róng, 026
rú yì cǎo, 051
Rú Yì Xǐ Jì, 051

S

Sān Bái Yǐn, 065, 066
sāng bái pí, 021, 027, 040, 042, 094, 171
Sāng Bái Pí Xǐ Fāng, 171
sāng jì shēng, 100, 176
sāng shèn, 083, 096, 099, 101, 107, 109, 176, 183
sāng yè, 019, 107, 172
Sān Huáng Shí Gāo Tāng, 044
sān léng, 030
Sargassum, 019, 024, 029, 204
Scolopendra, 141
Semen Armeniacae Amarum, 020
Semen Astragali Complanati, 176
Semen Cassiae, 144
Semen Coicis, 164, 203
Semen Cuscutae, 083, 101, 166
Semen Dolichoris Lablab, 046
Semen Ginkgo, 017, 056
Semen Juglandis, 145, 176
Semen Momordicae, 208
Semen Nelumbinis, 096, 177
Semen Persicae, 029, 033, 081, 103
Semen Plantaginis, 179, 183
Semen Platycladi, 176
Semen Pruni, 030
Semen Sesami Nigrum, 098, 106, 111, 183
Semen Sinapis, 189
Semen Sojae Nigrum, 109
Semen Vaccariae, 014, 016, 171, 172, 178
Semen Ziziphi Spinosae, 096, 101
shān dòu gēn, 063
shān nài, 093
shān zhā, 013, 023, 026, 046, 201
shān zhī zǐ, 106
shān zhū yú, 124, 166
shā yuàn jí lí, 176
shé chuáng zǐ, 093
shēng dì huáng, 010, 012, 021, 023, 024, 026, 028, 029, 083, 106, 107, 162, 183
shēng hé shǒu wū, 023, 026, 029
shēng jiāng, 091, 117, 131, 147, 173
shēng má, 044
shēng mù biē, 208
shēng shān zhā, 030
shēng shí gāo, 021, 027
Shēn Líng Bái Zhú Powder, 136
Shén Yìng Yǎng Zhēn Dān, 133
shí gāo, 048
Shí Quán Dà Bǔ Gāo, 087
shú dì huáng, 099, 101, 102, 104, 106, 124, 134, 180
shuǐ niú jiǎo, 043
Sì Huáng Gāo, 017, 034
Sì Jūn Zǐ Tāng, 134, 194
Sì Wù Tāng, 041, 083
Spica Prunellae, 024, 041
Spina Gleditsiae, 012, 171, 193
Squama Manis, 012
suān zǎo rén, 096, 101
Sulfur, 202

T

tài zǐ shēn, 107, 110, 195

Táo Hóng Sì Wù Tāng, 011, 032, 041, 042
táo rén, 029, 033, 081, 103
Thallus Laminariae, 019, 024, 029, 204
tiān huā fěn, 023, 029
tiān má, 142
Tōng Qiào Huó Xuè Tāng, 112, 136
tòu gǔ cǎo, 094, 171, 193
Tòu Gǔ Cǎo Fāng, 171
tǔ fú líng, 011, 101, 196
Tuō Fà Zài Shēng Jì, 172
tù sī zǐ, 083, 101, 166

V

Vitamin A, 175

W

wáng bù liú xíng, 014, 016, 171, 172, 178
wǔ bèi zǐ, 171
Wū Fà Shēng Fà Dīng, 092, 122, 205
wú gōng, 141
Wú Gōng Oil, 173
Wǔ Wèi Qīng Dú Yǐn, 040
Wǔ Wèi Xiāo Dú Yǐn, 040, 044
wǔ wèi zǐ, 101
wǔ zhuǎ lóng, 109

X

xià kū cǎo, 024, 041

xiāng bái zhǐ, 173
xiāng fù, 041, 082, 143
Xiāng Jú Jiǔ, 173
xiān líng pí, 198
xiān máo, 198
Xiāo Chuāng Měi Róng Tāng, 040
Xiāo Cuò Líng, 056
Xiāo Cuò Líng Dīng, 064
Xiāo Cuò Miàn Mó, 057
Xiāo Cuò Tāng, 010, 011, 013, 034, 040
Xiāo Cuò Yǐn, 040, 053
Xiāo Fēng Sǎn, 057
Xiāo Shī Sǎn, 055
Xiè Bái Sǎn, 040
Xiè Xīn Tāng, 043
Xǐ Liǎn Měi Róng Tāng, 018
xìng rén, 177
xī yáng shēn, 092
xuán shēn, 023, 026, 083, 107

Y

Yǎng Xuè Shēng Fà Tāng, 145
Yǎng Yīn Qīng Fèi Tāng, 136
yè jiāo téng, 092, 104
yě jú huā, 040, 171
yì mǔ cǎo, 026, 064, 204
Yì Mǔ Shèng Jīn Dān, 032
yīn chén, 164, 196
yīn chén hāo, 022, 042

Yīn Chén Hāo Tāng, 040, 042
yín yáng huò, 026, 144, 189
yì yǐ rén, 164, 203
yuán huā, 113
yù jīn, 012, 014, 143, 203
yù lǐ rén, 030
Yùn Pí Sàn Jié Tāng, 046
Yù Nǚ Jiān, 045
yú xīng cǎo, 012, 013

Z

Zanthoxylum Bungeanum Mazim, 063
zào jiǎo cì, 012, 171, 193
zǎo xiū, 024
zé xiè, 010, 164, 179, 183
Zhī Bǎi Bā Wèi Wán, 040
Zhī Bǎi Dì Huáng Wán, 014, 035
zhì fù zǐ, 189
zhì hé shǒu wū, 079, 085, 147, 165, 166
zhī ma, 098
zhī mǔ, 010
Zhǐ Yǎng Shēng Fà Dīng, 205
Zhī Yì Xǐ Fāng, 171
zhī zǐ, 029
zhū líng, 179
Zī Fàng Tāng, 215
zǐ hé chē, 198
zǐ huā dì dīng, 027, 040, 063

General Index

A

accumulated heat in the lung and stomach, 029
acne, 005
acne associated with lung and stomach accumulated heat, 021
AH6a, 089, 169
Aloe, 043
alopecia totalis, 075, 076
alopecia universalis, 075
Alumen, 048, 093, 171, 178
Alumen dehydratum, 193
anxiety, 075
Arillus Longan, 177
Armeniacae Semen Amarum, 177
AT4, 016
atrophic scar, 024
auricular needle-embedding therapy, 016
aversion to cold, 078

B

bǎi bù, 063, 173
bái fán, 171
bái guǒ, 017
bái guǒ rén, 056
bǎi hé, 096, 177
Bái Hǔ Tāng, 032
bái huā shé shé cǎo, 018, 022, 026, 030
bái jí lí, 064
bái jiāng cán, 041
bái jiè zǐ, 189
bái sháo, 014, 081, 083, 104, 196
bái xiān pí, 162, 164, 196
bái zhǐ, 052
bái zhú, 085, 101, 164, 179, 183, 184
bǎi zǐ rén, 176
bān máo, 093, 139, 142, 173
Bān Tū Wán, 086
bàn xià, 092
běi xìng rén, 020
bì xiè, 164, 179
biǎn dòu, 046
Bīng Fà Shēng Zhǎng Fāng, 172
bīng piàn, 048
BL 17, 088
BL 18, 088, 090
BL 2, 015
BL 23, 088, 090

blackhead, 027, 031
blood and essence deficiency, 098
blood deficiency, 132
blood deficiency and wind dryness, 192, 213
blood deficiency with wind dryness, 209, 211
blood heat, 039, 087
blood heat and wind dryness, 161, 162, 208, 210
blood heat engendering wind, 077
blood heat in the lung and stomach channels, 008
blood stasis, 029, 079, 087, 135
blurred vision, 084
Bombyx Batryticatus, 041, 196
Borneolum, 018
Borneolum Syntheticum, 048
Bǔ Gān Tāng, 213
bǔ gǔ zhī, 124
Bulbus Lilii, 096, 177

C

Cacumen Platycladi, 030, 050, 093, 096, 147, 171, 173, 193, 199, 202
Calamina, 018
Camellia sinensis O. Ktze, 030
cāng ěr zǐ, 171, 172, 178
cāng zhú, 057
Cannabis Folium, 172, 174, 200
cǎo wū, 141
Caulis Impatientis, 094, 171, 193
Caulis Polygoni Multiflori, 092, 104
Caulis Spatholobi, 109
cè bǎi yè, 030, 050, 093, 096, 147, 171, 173, 193, 199, 202
chá shù gēn, 030
chái hú, 013, 014, 043, 081
Chái Hú Shū Gān Sǎn, 212
Chái Hú Shū Gān Tāng, 013
chán tuì, 027, 162
chǎo é zhú, 029
chǎo sān léng, 029
chē qián cǎo, 055
chē qián zǐ, 179, 183
chén pí, 082, 105
chest and rib-side pain, 082
chest distress, 080
chì sháo, 021, 024, 028, 029, 083
chì shí zhī, 179
chóng lóu, 063
Chú Zhī Shēng Fà Tāng, 217
chuān liàn zǐ, 203
chuān shān jiǎ, 012
chuān xiōng, 041, 081, 104, 183, 184
cí shí, 084
clear heat, 162
clear heat and cool the blood, 024
clear the lung and resolve toxins, 009
CO10, 089
CO14, 016, 089, 169
CO18, 015, 089
Colla Cornus Cervi, 134, 189
Concha Ostreae, 096, 196
congealing yin cold, 188
constipation, 011, 097
cool blood, 162
cool blood and extinguish wind, 082
Cordyceps, 093
Cornu Bubali, 043
Cornu Cervi, 189
Cortex Dictamni, 162, 164, 196
Cortex Eucommiae, 176
Cortex Lycii, 041
Cortex Mori, 021, 027, 040, 042, 094, 171
Cortex Moutan, 024, 028, 083, 106
cuán zhú, 015
Cuò Chuāng Gāo, 066
Cuò Chuāng Píng, 022, 040
Cuò Chuāng Qīng Xiāo Yǐn, 047
Cuò Chuāng Yǐn, 040
Cuò Líng Dīng, 016
Cuò Líng Shuāng, 016
Cuò Yù Sǎn, 050
cyst, 005, 030
cystic acne, 024

D

dōng chóng xià cǎo, 093
dōng qīng zǐ, 106
dà huáng, 011, 174
dà qīng yè, 042
dà zǎo, 177
dài zhě shí, 080, 174
damp-heat in the lung and stomach, 042
damp obstruction, 168
damp-heat, 163, 191, 192, 194, 196
damp-heat accumulating upwards, 209, 210
damp-heat accumulation, 213
damp-heat in the intestine and stomach, 044
damp-heat in the spleen and stomach, 161
dampness, 164
dampness accumulation due to spleen

deficiency, 212
dampness predominating over heat, 031
dān shēn, 010, 012, 026, 029, 030, 035, 197, 204
Dān Zhī Xiāo Yáo Sǎn, 032, 040
Dān Zhī Xiāo Yáo Wán, 015
dàn zhú yè, 043
dāng guī, 026, 081, 103, 104, 109, 123, 144, 162, 192
Dāng Guī Lú Huì Wán, 043
Dāng Guī Piàn, 087
dāng guī wěi, 050
dǎng shēn, 085
delayed menstruation, 026, 036
Dens Dragonis, 196
depressed internal fire, 105
dì fū zǐ, 030, 050, 196
dì gǔ pí, 041
dì huáng, 109
dì yú, 063
Diān Dǎo Sǎn, 055
disharmony of the penetrating and conception vessels, 008, 013, 036
dispel wind, 162
disperse phlegm and soften hardness, 024
dissipate cold, 189

distending pain in the breasts, 013
distending pain in the chest and hypochondria, 203
dizziness, 078, 084
drain fire, 009
dream-disturbed sleep, 009, 011
dry Moschus, 051
dry mouth, 162
dryness-heat, 031
DU 19, 087
DU 20, 087, 090, 169
DU 23, 087
dù zhòng, 176
dual deficiencies of qi and blood, 077
dusky purple tongue, 080

E

é zhú, 064
ear acupuncture, 089
ear apex, 015
early menstruation, 014
eliminate dampness, 183
endocrine, 015
enrich yin and drain fire, 009
Èr Chén Tāng, 041
Èr Xiān Tāng, 032
Èr Zhì Wán, 035, 040, 083, 111, 168
Eucalyptus robusta Sm, 051
even supplementation and

drainage, 015
EX-HN 3, 090
EX-HN 1, 169
exuberant lung-stomach heat, 011
exuberant wind, 168

F

fáng fēng, 056, 162
fatigue, 197
fēi gān shí, 018
Fěn Cì Jiān, 047
five-center heat, 163
flaky alopecia, 082
Flos Albiziae, 143
Flos Carthami, 012, 029, 033, 081, 098, 103, 139, 173
Flos Celosiae Cristatae, 101
Flos Chrysanthemi, 027, 162
Flos Chrysanthemi Indici, 040, 171
Flos Genkwa, 113
Flos Lonicerae Japonicae, 040
Flos Rhododendri Mollis, 143
Flos Rosae Rugosae, 055
Folium Eriobotryae, 021, 027, 028, 040
Folium Isatidis, 042
Folium Mori, 019, 107, 172
fortify the spleen and benefit qi, 084

Fructus Cannabis, 030
Fructus Chaenomelis, 099
Fructus Cnidii, 093
Fructus Corni, 124, 166
Fructus Crataegi, 013, 023, 026, 046, 201
Fructus Forsythiae, 040
Fructus Gardeniae, 029, 106
Fructus Hordei Germinatus, 205
Fructus Jujubae, 177
Fructus Kochiae, 030, 050, 196
Fructus Ligustri Lucidi, 010, 012, 014, 029, 041, 097, 100, 166, 183, 195
Fructus Liquidambaris, 180
Fructus Lycii, 079, 099, 100, 102, 111, 166
Fructus Mori, 083, 096, 099, 101, 107, 109, 176, 183
Fructus Psoraleae, 124
Fructus Rosae Laevigatae, 187
Fructus Rubi, 176
Fructus Schisandrae Chinensis, 101
Fructus Toosendan, 203
Fructus Tribuli, 064, 162
Fructus Trichosanthis, 065
Fructus Viticis, 187
Fructus Xanthii, 171, 172, 178

Fù Fāng Shé Cǎo Tāng, 065
fú líng, 079, 085, 164
Fú Líng Wán, 045
fù pén zǐ, 176
fullness and oppression in the chest and abdomen, 105

G

Galla Chinensis, 171
gān dì huáng, 176
gān sōng, 173
gān shè xiāng, 051
gān suì, 113
GB 20, 087, 090
ghost-shaved head, 076
ghost shaving head, 133
ghost-licked head, 076, 131
glossy scalp wind, 076, 133, 134
gǒu qǐ zǐ, 079, 099, 100, 102, 111, 166
Gù Shèn Shēng Fà Tāng, 099
gǔ suì bǔ, 093, 140
guì zhī, 189
Guì Zhī Jiā Sháo Yào Tāng, 190
Gypsum Fibrosum, 021, 027, 048

H

Haematitum, 080, 174
Hǎi Ài Tāng, 133
hǎi zǎo, 019, 024, 029, 204

hair loss, 078
Halloysitum Rubrum, 179
hàn lián cǎo, 010, 012, 014, 041, 091, 166
hé huān huā, 143
hé shǒu wū, 092, 099, 103, 123, 176, 180
Hé Shǒu Wū Kǔ Shēn Hé Jì, 052
hé táo rén, 145, 176
headache, 080
heart and liver Fire, 043
heat induced by blood deficiency, 086
heat predominating over dampness, 031
hēi dòu, 109
hēi zhī ma, 106, 111, 183
henry chloranthus, 093
Herba Artemisiae Scopariae, 022, 042, 164, 196
Herba Cistanches, 026
Herba Ecliptae, 010, 014, 041, 091, 139, 147, 166
Herba Epimedii, 026, 144, 189, 198
Herba Eupatorii, 192
Herba Hedyotis Diffusae, 018, 022, 026, 030, 196
Herba Houttuyniae, 012, 013
Herba Leonuri, 026, 064, 204
Herba Lophatheri, 043
Herba Plantaginis, 055

Herba Portulacae, 054
Herba Schizonepetae, 050, 056, 162
Herba Taraxaci, 012, 013, 024, 040, 064, 099
Herba Taxilli, 100, 176
Herba Violae, 027, 040, 063
hóng huā, 012, 029, 033, 081, 098, 103, 139, 173
hǔ zhàng, 022, 026, 030, 063
huā jiāo, 131, 134, 140, 173
Huà Yū Sàn Jié Wán, 028
huái niú xī, 124
huáng dān, 018
huáng jīng, 109, 166
huáng lián, 174
Huáng Lián Jiě Dú Tāng, 040
huáng qí, 085, 102, 145, 192, 195, 197
Huáng Qí Jiàng Zhōng Tāng, 134
huáng qín, 021, 027, 174
huǒ má rén, 030
Huó Xuè Shēng Fà Yǐn, 217
HX6, 015
hyperactivity of fire due to yin deficiency, 029

I

Ilicis Chinensis Semen, 106
infection, 114
insomnia, 075, 078, 080, 084, 088, 097, 101, 165, 196, 203
insufficiency of the liver and kidney, 077, 100
invigorate the blood and dispel stasis, 030
irregular menstruation, 013
irritability, 080, 097
itching, 088

J

jī guān huā, 101
jí lí, 162
jī xuè téng, 109
jiá chē, 015
Jiā Wèi Sì Wù Tāng, 144
Jiā Wèi Xiāo Yáo Sǎn, 043
Jiàn Pí Wán, 168
jiāng cán, 196
jiāo mù, 063
Jiě Dú Huà Yū Tāng, 053
Jié Fū Yǐn, 216
Jīn Huáng Gāo, 034
Jīn Huáng Sǎn, 050
Jīn Jú Xiāng Jiān Jì, 065
jīn sù lán, 093
jīn yín huā, 040
Jīn Yín Huā Tāng, 055
jīn yīng zǐ, 187
jīng jiè, 050, 056, 162
jú huā, 027, 162
jú pí, 041
jué míng zǐ, 144

K

Kè Tū Níng Dīng, 147

KI 3, 088
kidney deficiency with blood dryness, 212
kidney yin deficiency, 007, 176
kū fán, 048, 193
kǔ shēn, 030, 050, 162, 171, 178, 180
kūn bù, 019, 024, 029, 204

L

Lantana camara, 051
lethargy, 084
lián qiào, 040
Lián Shí Sǎn, 051
lián zǐ, 096, 177
Liáng Xuè Xiāo Fēng Sǎn, 162
líng líng xiāng, 173
liú huáng, 202
Liù Wèi Dì Huáng Wán, 168, 194
liver and kidney are of the same source, 035
liver and kidney deficiency, 102, 108, 165, 168, 209, 210, 211, 213
liver and kidney yin deficiency, 105
liver constraint and blood deficiency, 181
liver constraint and qi stagnation, 015
liver constraint transforming into fire, 082
liver depression and blood

stasis, 077
lóng chǐ, 196
lóng dăn căo, 043
Lóng Dăn Xiè Gān Tāng, 040
Lóng Dăn Xiè Gān Wán, 168
lóng yăn ròu, 177
LR 3, 087
lú huì, 043
lù jiăo jiāo, 134, 189
lù jiăo piàn, 189
lù lù tōng, 180
lung and stomach accumulated heat, 027
lung heat, 034, 042, 043
lung qi deficiency, 177
lung wind, 028
lung wind acne, 006
lung yin deficiency, 177

M

mă chǐ xiàn, 054
má yè, 172, 174, 200
Magnetitum, 084
mài dōng, 023, 029
mài yá, 205
màn jīng zǐ, 187
Máo Fà Chōng Jì, 215
méi guī huā, 055
Méi Huā Diăn Shé Wán, 015
méi piàn, 018
míng fán, 093, 178
ministerial fire, 006
mò hàn lián, 139, 147
moisten dryness, 162, 185
mŭ dān pí, 021, 024, 028, 083, 106
mù guā, 099
mŭ lì, 096, 196
Mylabris, 093, 139, 142, 173

N

nào yáng huā, 143
nightmare, 080
niú xī, 079
nodule, 005, 022, 030
nourish blood, 104, 183
nourish liver and kidney, 078
nourish yin, 009, 105
nourish yin and clear heat, 011, 185
nǚ zhēn zǐ, 010, 012, 014, 029, 041, 097, 100, 166, 183, 195

O

oily dandruff, 203

P

palpitation, 084
paprika, 139
papule, 005, 025
pèi lán, 192
Pericarpium Citri Reticulatae, 041, 082, 105
Pericarpium Zanthoxyli, 131, 134, 140, 173
Periostracum Cicadae, 027, 162
pessimism, 095
phlegm and blood stasis binding together, 008
phlegm dampness with stasis heat, 211
phlegm stasis, 028
phlegm, heat and stasis binding, 019
Pí Pá Qīng Fèi Yǐn, 021, 028, 032, 040, 041, 042
pí pá yè, 021, 027, 028, 040
Pí Zhī Cā Jì, 172
Píng Cuò Tāng, 023
Placenta Hominis, 198
plum-blossom needling, 089, 170
Polyporus, 179
poor appetite, 088
poor memory, 165
Poria, 079, 085, 164
postpartum hemorrhaging, 121
profuse dreaming, 196
pú gōng yīng, 012, 013, 024, 040, 064, 099
Pŭ Jì Xiāo Dú Yǐn, 046
purge fire, 105
pustule, 005, 022, 024, 027, 030

Q

qi and blood deficiency, 100, 102
Qī Băo Měi Rán Dān, 078,

086, 166
qi deficiency, 197
Qǐ Jú Dì Huáng Wán, 087
qi stagnation and blood stasis, 042, 203
qiāng huó, 111
Qīng Fèi Qū Zhī Fāng, 066
Qīng Fèi Xiāo Dú Yǐn, 040
Qīng Rè Huà Yū Xiāo Chuāng Sǎn, 053
Qīng Wèi Sǎn, 044
Qīng Yíng Tāng, 043
Qū Shī Jiàn Fà Tāng, 216
Qù Zhī Chōng Jì, 215
Qū Zhī Shēng Fà Dīng, 205
quán guā lóu, 065

R

Radix Achyranthis Bidentatae, 079, 124
Radix Aconiti Kusnezoffii, 141
Radix Aconiti Lateralis Praeparata, 189
Radix Angelicae Dahuricae, 052, 173, 203
Radix Angelicae Sinensis, 026, 050, 081, 103, 104, 109, 123, 144, 162, 192
Radix Astragali, 085, 102, 145, 192, 195, 197
Radix Bupleuri, 013, 014, 043, 081
Radix Codonopsis, 085
Radix Curcumae, 012, 014, 143, 203
Radix et Rhizoma Nardostachyos, 173
Radix et Rhizoma Rhei, 011, 174
Radix et Rhizoma Salviae Miltiorrhizae, 010, 012, 026, 029, 030, 035, 197, 204
Radix et Rhizoma Sophorae Tonkinensis, 063
Radix Gentianae, 043
Radix Ginseng, 173
Radix Ipomoeae Cairicae, 109
Radix Kansui, 113
Radix Ophiopogonis, 023, 029
Radix Paeoniae Alba, 014, 081, 083, 104, 196
Radix Paeoniae Rubra, 021, 024, 028, 029, 083
Radix Panacis Quinquefolii, 092
Radix Polygoni multiflori, 023, 026, 029
Radix Polygoni Multiflori, 092, 099, 103, 123, 176, 180
Radix Polygoni Multiflori Praeparata cum Succo Glycines Sotae, 079, 085, 147, 165, 166
Radix Pseudostellariae, 107, 110, 195
Radix Rehmanniae, 010, 012, 021, 023, 024, 026, 028, 029, 083, 106, 107, 109, 162, 176, 183
Radix Rehmanniae Praeparata, 099, 101, 102, 104, 106, 124, 134, 180
Radix Sanguisorbae, 063
Radix Saposhnikoviae, 056, 162
Radix Scrophulariae, 023, 026, 083, 107
Radix Scutellariae, 021, 027, 174
Radix Sophorae Flavescentis, 030, 050, 162, 178, 180
Radix Stemonae, 063, 173
Radix Trichosanthis, 023, 029
Ramulus Cinnamomi, 189
raw Fructus Crataegi, 030
reduce swelling and expel pus, 012
relieve itching, 185
rén shēn, 173
Rén Shēn Yǎng Róng Tāng, 085
Rén Shēn Yǎng Róng Wán, 086
resolve toxins, 027
restlessness, 080, 097
Rhizoma Alismatis, 010, 164, 179, 183
Rhizoma Anemarrhenae, 010
Rhizoma Atractylodis, 057
Rhizoma Atractylodis

Macrocephalae, 085, 101, 179, 183, 184
Rhizoma Atractylodis Macrocephalae (dry-fried), 164
Rhizoma Chuanxiong, 041, 081, 104, 183, 184
Rhizoma Cimicifugae, 044
Rhizoma Coptidis, 174
Rhizoma Curculiginis, 198
Rhizoma Curcumae, 064
Rhizoma Curcumae (dry-fried), 029
Rhizoma Cyperi, 041, 082, 143
Rhizoma Dioscoreae Hypoglaucae, 164, 179
Rhizoma Drynariae, 093, 140
Rhizoma et Radix Notopterygii, 111
Rhizoma Gastrodiae, 142
Rhizoma Kaempferiae, 093
Rhizoma Paridis, 024, 063
Rhizoma Pinelliae, 092
Rhizoma Polygonati, 109, 166
Rhizoma Polygoni Cuspidati, 022, 026, 030, 063
Rhizoma Smilacis Glabrae, 011, 101, 196
Rhizoma Sparganii, 030
Rhizoma Sparganii (dry-fried), 029

Rhizoma Zingiberis Recens, 091, 117, 131, 147, 173
ròu cōng róng, 026
rú yì cǎo, 051
Rú Yì Xǐ Jì, 051

S

Sān Bái Yǐn, 065, 066
Sān Huáng Shí Gāo Tāng, 044
sān léng, 030
sāng bái pí, 021, 027, 040, 042, 094, 171
Sāng Bái Pí Xǐ Fāng, 171
sāng jì shēng, 100, 176
sāng shèn, 083, 096, 099, 101, 107, 109, 176, 183
sāng yè, 019, 107, 172
Sargassum, 019, 024, 029, 204
scalp itchiness, 162
scalp self-massage, 090
Scolopendra, 141
seborrheic dermatitis, 171
sebum secretions, 201
Semen Armeniacae Amarum, 020
Semen Astragali Complanati, 176
Semen Cassiae, 144
Semen Coicis, 164, 203
Semen Cuscutae, 083, 101, 166
Semen Dolichoris Lablab, 046

Semen Ginkgo, 017, 056
Semen Juglandis, 145, 176
Semen Momordicae, 208
Semen Nelumbinis, 096, 177
Semen Persicae, 029, 033, 081, 103
Semen Plantaginis, 179, 183
Semen Platycladi, 176
Semen Pruni, 030
Semen Sesami Nigrum, 098, 106, 111, 183
Semen Sinapis, 189
Semen Sojae Nigrum, 109
Semen Vaccariae, 014, 016, 171, 172, 178
Semen Ziziphi Spinosae, 096, 101
seminal emission, 078
shā yuàn jí lí, 176
shān dòu gēn, 063
shān nài, 093
shān zhā, 013, 023, 026, 046, 201
shān zhī zǐ, 106
shān zhū yú, 124, 166
shé chuáng zǐ, 093
Shēn Líng Bái Zhú Powder, 136
Shén Yìng Yǎng Zhēn Dān, 133
shēng dì huáng, 010, 012, 021, 023, 024, 026, 028, 029, 083, 106, 107, 162, 183

Shēng Fà Dīng, 173
Shēng Fà Jiǔ, 173
Shēng Fà Tāng, 214
Shēng Fà Wán, 086, 216
shēng hé shǒu wū, 023, 026, 029
shēng jiāng, 091, 117, 131, 147, 173
shēng má, 044
shēng mù biē, 208
shēng shān zhā, 030
shēng shí gāo, 021, 027
shí gāo, 048
Shí Quán Dà Bǔ Gāo, 087
shú dì huáng, 099, 101, 102, 104, 106, 124, 134, 180
shuǐ niú jiǎo, 043
Sì Huáng Gāo, 017, 034
Sì Jūn Zǐ Tāng, 134, 194
Sì Wù Tāng, 041, 083
SJ 17, 169
somnolence, 084
soreness and weakness of the lower back and knees, 165
sorrow, 095
SP 10, 087, 088, 090
SP 6, 087, 088, 090
Spica Prunellae, 024, 041
Spina Gleditsiae, 012, 171, 193
spleen deficiency leading to damp encumbrance, 181
spleen-stomach disharmony, 101
spontaneous sweating, 197
Squama Manis, 012
ST 36, 087
ST 6, 015
ST 7, 015
ST 8, 169
stabbing pain on the scalp, 080
strengthen the spleen, 164, 183
stress, 095
suān zǎo rén, 096, 101
subcortex, 016
Sulfur, 202

T

Tōng Qiào Huó Xuè Tāng, 112, 136
tài zǐ shēn, 107, 110, 195
tanshinone, 197
Táo Hóng Sì Wù Tāng, 011, 032, 041, 042
táo rén, 029, 033, 081, 103
TF4, 089
Thallus Laminariae, 019, 024, 029, 204
thin falling hair, 163
thirst, 097
tian gui, 006, 007
tiān huā fěn, 023, 029
tiān má, 142
tinnitus, 078
tonify qi to produce blood, 197
tonify the liver and kidney, 104, 165
tòu gǔ cǎo, 094, 171, 193
Tòu Gǔ Cǎo Fāng, 171
transform stasis and dissipate nodules, 011
tǔ fú líng, 011, 101, 196
tù sī zǐ, 083, 101, 166
Tuō Fà Zài Shēng Jì, 172

V

vertigo, 078
vexation, 009
Vitamin A, 175

W

wáng bù liú xíng, 014, 016, 171, 172, 178
warm yang, 189
weak nutritive qi and strong defensive qi, 190
whitehead, 031
wind dryness, 171
wind dryness due to blood deficiency, 101
wind heat in the lung channel, 042
wǔ bèi zǐ, 171
Wū Fà Shēng Fà Dīng, 092, 122, 205
wú gōng, 141
Wǔ Wèi Qīng Dú Yǐn, 040
Wǔ Wèi Xiāo Dú Yǐn, 040, 044
wǔ wèi zǐ, 101
wǔ zhuǎ lóng, 109

X

Xǐ Liǎn Měi Róng Tāng, 018
xī yáng shēn, 092
xià guān, 015
xià kū cǎo, 024, 041
xiān líng pí, 198
xiān máo, 198
xiāng bái zhǐ, 173
xiāng fù, 041, 082, 143
Xiāng Jú Jiǔ, 173
Xiāo Chuāng Měi Róng Tāng, 040
Xiāo Cuò Líng, 056
Xiāo Cuò Líng Dīng, 064
Xiāo Cuò Miàn Mó, 057
Xiāo Cuò Sǎn, 017
Xiāo Cuò Tāng, 010, 011, 013, 034, 040
Xiāo Cuò Yǐn, 040, 053
Xiāo Fēng Sǎn, 057
Xiāo Shī Sǎn, 055
Xiè Bái Sǎn, 040
Xiè Xīn Tāng, 043
xìng rén, 177

xuán shēn, 023, 026, 083, 107

Y

yang qi deficiency, 188
Yǎng Xuè Shēng Fà Tāng, 145
Yǎng Yīn Qīng Fèi Tāng, 136
yè jiāo téng, 092, 104
yě jú huā, 040, 171
yì mǔ cǎo, 026, 064, 204
Yì Mǔ Shèng Jīn Dān, 032
yì yǐ rén, 164, 203
yīn chén, 164, 196
yīn chén hāo, 022, 042
Yīn Chén Hāo Tāng, 040, 042
yin deficiency generating internal heat, 009, 020
yin essence deficiency, 191, 198
yín yáng huò, 026, 144, 189
yù jīn, 012, 014, 143, 203
yù lǐ rén, 030
Yù Nǚ Jiān, 045
yú xīng cǎo, 012, 013
yuán huā, 113
Yùn Pí Sàn Jié Tāng, 046

Z

Zanthoxylum Bungeanum Mazim, 063
zào jiāo cì, 012, 171, 193
zǎo xiū, 024
zé xiè, 010, 164, 179, 183
Zhī Bǎi Bā Wèi Wán, 040
Zhī Bǎi Dì Huáng Wán, 014, 035
zhì fù zǐ, 189
zhì hé shǒu wū, 079, 085, 147, 165, 166
zhī ma, 098
zhī mǔ, 010
Zhǐ Yǎng Shēng Fà Dīng, 205
Zhī Yì Xǐ Fāng, 171
zhī zǐ, 029
zhū líng, 179
Zī Fàng Tāng, 215
zǐ hé chē, 198
zǐ huā dì dīng, 027, 040, 063

Notes

图书在版编目（CIP）数据

中医临床实用系列：痤疮与脱发（英文）/范瑞强主编.
—北京：人民卫生出版社，2008.4
ISBN 978-7-117-09888-5

Ⅰ.中… Ⅱ.范… Ⅲ.①痤疮—中医治疗法—英文②脱发—中医治疗法—英文 Ⅳ.R275.987

中国版本图书馆 CIP 数据核字（2008）第 033559 号

中医临床实用系列：痤疮与脱发（英文）

主　　编：范瑞强
出版发行：人民卫生出版社（中继线 +8610-6761-6688）
地　　址：中国北京市丰台区方庄芳群园三区 3 号楼
邮　　编：100078
网　　址：http://www.pmph.com
E - mail：pmph @ pmph.com
发　　行：pmphsales@gmail.com
购书热线：+8610-6769-1034（电话及传真）
开　　本：787×1092　1/16
版　　次：2008年4月第1版　2008年4月第1版第一次印刷
标准书号：ISBN 978-7-117-09888-5/R·9889

版权所有，侵权必究，打击盗版举报电话：**+8610-8761-3394**
（凡属印装质量问题请与本社销售部联系退换）